he

OSCE

ery, UK

JS
ery, UK

spital,

Foreword by

MAURICE HAWTHORNE
Consultant Otolaryngologist
James Cook University Hospital, Middlesborough
Director of Education, ENT UK

Radcliffe Publishing
London • New York

Radcliffe Publishing Ltd
33–41 Dallington Street
London
EC1V 0BB
United Kingdom

www.radcliffepublishing.com

British Library Cataloguing in Publication Data

A catalogue record for this book is available from the British Library.

ISBN-13: 978 184619 572 3

The paper used for the text pages of this book is FSC® certified. FSC (The Forest Stewardship Council®) is an international network to promote responsible management of the world's forests.

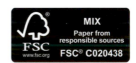

Typeset by Darkriver Design, Auckland, New Zealand
Printed and bound by Hobbs the Printers, Totton, Hants, UK

Contents

Foreword

It is with great pleasure that I write this Foreword. In 2001, I was asked to undertake a review of the DLO examination which was founded by Sir William Milligan, former head of the department at Manchester Royal Infirmary where I was house man in 1977. In 1923, seven years before his death, Sir William was the prime mover at The Royal College of Surgeons of England for the introduction of a specific examination and qualification for Ear, Nose and Throat Surgeons. After the introduction of the FRCS in ENT after the Second World War, the popularity of the DLO began to wane. In 2001, it was clear that the examination had had its day and so was abolished. There was some debate at the time as to whether something new should replace the DLO.

Out of these meetings the DO-HNS was born. It was clear that the design of the old DLO did not meet modern educational assessment standards. In the latter years of the last century debate had been heated in the Court of Examiners over introduction of an OSCE style examination in the MRCS with the status quo being consistently maintained throughout this period. Derek Skinner, Adrian Drake-Lee and I pushed for the introduction of an OSCE style examination and this was adopted by the Board. The result was an MCQ examination followed by an OSCE, the format which still survives today.

In many ways whilst examination and assessment has moved significantly in the last decade, learning material is just beginning to catch up. This book is part of that renaissance of learning techniques. I thoroughly recommend it to all those who are preparing themselves for OSCE examinations in Otolaryngology.

Maurice Hawthorne
Consultant Otolaryngologist
James Cook University Hospital, Middlesborough
Director of Education, ENT UK
December 2011

Preface

This book was born out of the real absence of a suitable revision guide while preparing for the Diploma of Otolaryngology – Head and Neck Surgery (DO-HNS) exam ourselves. While studying, we took careful notes of what would have been useful to us in an all-encompassing revision guide and, after the exam, we looked back at which parts of our revision were fruitful in helping us pass.

The DO-HNS OSCE examination has recently been made a route to gaining Membership of the Royal College of Surgeons (MRCS). This book covers all aspects of the DO-HNS and MRCS (ENT) OSCE, particularly the examination, communication and picture stations. We have purposely followed the format of the exam, giving the reader a real advantage in passing what is now a requirement for progression to registrar training in otolaryngology (ENT). This book will be useful for current ENT and surgical trainees and those wishing to refresh their knowledge of common ENT problems, including general practitioners with a special interest in ENT. In addition to its function as an exam preparation guide, this book will also act as a valuable quick reference in any ENT clinic or treatment room. It will also be a helpful resource for medical students undertaking their ENT attachment and in the preparation for their final examinations, which routinely feature ENT-based OSCE stations.

We offer you this book with the confidence that it adds something new and useful to the bookshelf of every budding otolaryngologist, and wish you the very best when sitting your exam.

Joe Manjaly
Peter Kullar
December 2011

About the authors

Peter Kullar is an Academic Clinical Fellow in ENT in the Northern Deanery. He graduated from Cambridge University and has successfully obtained full MRCS and DO-HNS. He has a specialist interest in otology, particularly the application of stem cells and molecular therapies for hearing restoration.

Joseph Manjaly is a Core Surgical Trainee in ENT in the Wessex Deanery and is currently National Core Trainee Representative for the Association of Otolaryngologists in Training. After gaining a first class intercalated BSc in Physiology, he graduated with his year group's highest Foundation Programme application score and has worked as an anatomy demonstrator at Bristol University.

Philip Yates is a Consultant ENT Surgeon at the Freeman Hospital, Newcastle upon Tyne, and an Associate Clinical Lecturer at Newcastle University. He has an interest in both undergraduate and postgraduate education in ENT. He has organised a successful revision course for the Intercollegiate Specialty Examination in Otolaryngology since 2003. He has been an OSCE examiner both for undergraduate exams and for the DO-HNS examination.

Acknowledgements

- Oliver Dale, ENT Registrar, Oxford Deanery
- Leanna Norris, Audiologist, Salisbury District Hospital
- Timothy Biggs, Core Surgical Trainee, Wessex Deanery
- Rachel Mackinnon, Foundation Year 2, Wessex Deanery
- Simon Mordecai, Core Surgical Trainee, Wessex Deanery
- Simon Dennis, Consultant ENT Surgeon, Salisbury District Hospital

Abbreviations

ACE	angiotensin-converting enzyme
ANCA	anti-neutrophil cytoplasmic antibody
AOAEs	automated otoacoustic emissions
AOM	acute otitis media
BIPP	bismuth, iodoform and paraffin paste
BPPV	benign paroxysmal positional vertigo
CBT	cognitive behavioural therapy
CNS	central nervous system
CS	Churg–Strauss syndrome
CSF	cerebrospinal fluid
CSOM	chronic suppurative otitis media
CT	computed tomography
CXR	chest X-ray
DO-HNS	Diploma of Otolaryngology – Head and Neck Surgery
EAC	external auditory canal
ENT	ear, nose and throat
ESR	erythrocyte sedimentation rate
FBC	full blood count
FNA	fine needle aspiration
FNE	flexible nasendoscopy
FOSIT	feeling of something in the throat
GP	general practitioner
GRBAS	grade, roughness, breathiness, asthenia, strain scale
HIV	human immunodeficiency virus
ICP	intracranial pressure
INR	international normalised ratio
JVP	jugular venous pulse
LMN	lower motor neuron
LPR	laryngopharyngeal reflux
MRCS	Membership of the Royal College of Surgeons
MRI	magnetic resonance imaging
OD	olfactory dysfunction

OE	otitis externa
OME	otitis media with effusion
OSCE	objective structured clinical examination
PNS	post-nasal space
PPI	proton-pump inhibitor
PTA	pure-tone audiometry
SCC	squamous cell carcinoma
SNHL	sensorineural hearing loss
ST3	Specialty Training Year 3
TB	tuberculosis
TM	tympanic membrane
TORCH	toxoplasmosis, other, rubella, cytomegalovirus, herpes simplex virus
U+Es	urea and electrolytes
UMN	upper motor neuron
URTI	upper respiratory tract infection
USS	ultrasound scan
WG	Wegener's granulomatosis

Richenda and Iqi Kullar
George and Sheeba Manjaly

The DO-HNS and MRCS (ENT) Examination and How to Pass It

The Diploma of Otolaryngology – Head and Neck Surgery (DO-HNS) has existed in one form or another since 2003, after replacing the old Diploma of Laryngology and Otology. Your reason for sitting the examination will most likely be as a route into higher ear, nose and throat (ENT) training or as a way of showing a special interest as part of general practice or allied specialty training. In recent years, DO-HNS became a requirement for entry to higher training in ENT and a core requirement for progression to the Specialty Training Year 3 (ST3) grade.

The examination still consists of two parts: Part 1, a 2-hour written paper comprising multiple-choice questions and extended matching questions, and Part 2, the objective structured clinical examination (OSCE) on which this book focuses. Initially, candidates for ENT ST3 tended to sit the full DO-HNS examination in addition to both parts of the regular Membership of the Royal College of Surgeons (MRCS) examination. The rules changed in 2008 to allow the dual award of an MRCS diploma in addition to the DO-HNS after passing DO-HNS Parts 1 and 2 plus MRCS Part A.

In May 2011, in order to address issues of equivalence, the regulations changed again, with a new 'MRCS (ENT)' being awarded to candidates passing MRCS Part A and the DO-HNS OSCE. The DO-HNS examination, in both parts, can still be sat as a stand-alone examination for those outside of ENT higher surgical training.

Be sure to get up to speed with the latest examination announcements and the core syllabus on the DO-HNS website (www.intercollegiatemrcs.org.uk/dohns).

We are confident that using this book will provide a firm grounding for passing the OSCE. While there is no longer a rule governing experience, time spent in an ENT job is invaluable, as many of the questions are designed to test 'on-the-job experience'. Both junior authors had at least 6 months' senior house officer experience before passing the examination.

The examination is held three times per year, rotating among London, Edinburgh and Glasgow, so be sure to register and pay fees in good time. The colleges are very strict on application deadlines and they tend not to make exceptions for late entries. It is a good idea to sort out travel and accommodation as early as possible, as the later these details are arranged, the more expensive they become.

Allow 2–3 months' preparation time alongside your normal clinical commitments. In addition to this book, you will find it useful to work through an ENT picture atlas and to selectively read a more comprehensive ENT textbook, of which there are many on the market.

The importance of the communication skills section of the examination must be stressed and many candidates tend to find this section problematic. For those who are not native English speakers or do not have a degree from a UK medical school, it may be appropriate to consider further training in communication skills. Most important, you must practise the examination and communication scenarios *ad nauseam*. In our experience, obliging friends and relatives can be bribed relatively cheaply. It may also be worthwhile attending a dedicated DO-HNS revision course. It is surprising how effectively a substantial financial outlay focuses the revision-weary mind!

You will find that the examination question style is similar to those in this book. At the time of writing, the OSCE consists of around 25 stations plus three to four rest stations, each lasting 7 minutes. Twenty of these stations are unmanned written stations. The examination lasts approximately 3½ hours, but with the added administration time it allows at least 6 hours door to door.

In the clinical examination stations, we ought to mention that you are not required to present your findings at the end of the examination. However, some candidates find the 'running commentary' approach helps them remember the pattern of their examination scheme. The examiner is there to make sure the question information is correctly presented to the candidate and to mark the station according to a structured scheme.

It is also important to note that the mark scheme for the written stations tends to accept short, succinct answers. Largely, time is in abundance for these stations. Do not feel you have to write long paragraphs. Often, a sentence or a few words will be enough to secure the marks. In our experience, for each question the number of lines given in the answer booklet corresponds with the number of marks available. For example, a question with four lines in the answer space means there are four possible marks to be picked up. We cannot stress enough how important it is that you read and re-read the question. It sounds obvious, but make sure you actually answer the question too! For example, if the question asks for four causes of something, you will be scored only for the first four that you list. This means if you list six causes and the first two are wrong, you will only score two marks, even if the next four are correct.

Be reassured that pass rates have tended to be between 45% and 75% in recent years. With some considered preparation this is an eminently passable and fair examination.

On a final note, as you can imagine, a 3½ hour examination is long and most certainly feels it. It is important to be rested before the examination. Some people find it useful to take a small snack with them to keep up those flagging blood sugar levels!

General tips for the communication and history stations

The communication stations are probably the most intimidating part of the examination. You are faced with an actor and an examiner. To those not familiar with the OSCE set-up this can be somewhat daunting. Staying calm and unflustered will be to your advantage. Be reassured that there are plenty of marks available for the simple things. It is vital to blind your mind to the contrived nature of the situation and treat the actor as a patient, as you would in clinical practice. Do not expect too much interaction from the examiner; it is normal for them to remain entirely passive. This can be a little disconcerting if you are looking for affirmation. Likewise, do not rely on the examiner for timekeeping. There will be no signal that the 7 minutes allotted for the station is coming to an end. It is well worth practising some of the scenarios in this book, to give you an idea of how best to manage the time effectively.

For all of the history stations it is useful to adopt the 'open to closed' question approach. Start general and then work on to the specifics of the presenting complaint. A useful general opener could be: 'Could you explain to me in your own words the symptoms that you have been experiencing?'

It is also useful to contextualise the patient's symptoms, so ask early on in the consultation about the effect of the symptoms on the patient's life. This is extremely important in the examination, as there are often marks for uncovering the patient's 'hidden agenda'. Being an examination, and hence by definition an artificial situation, you will find the actor's healthcare-seeking motivation tends to be rather more neatly constructed than in clinical practice. For example, the patient experiencing vertigo may have underlying concerns of a brain tumour, which they will reveal with some gentle, empathetic questioning. Uncovering the patients' **ICE** – **I**deas (as to aetiology), **C**oncerns (hidden agendas) and **E**xpectations (as to treatment and prognosis) – is a useful framework for establishing this vital narrative information.

Chapter 1 details a number of common ENT presentations and the best method for tackling them in the examination or in clinical practice. We have detailed a number of specific areas that will need to be explored in the consultations but it is important in each case that you start with general open questions. This will also help to establish a rapport with the patient, facilitating more specific questioning. Do remember that rapport, fluency and professionalism carry a lot of marks in the examination. Time is limited of course and it is also important to focus on the core symptoms and not be too distracted by interesting but fruitless tangential diversions.

CHAPTER 1

History Stations

There will be at least three history stations in the examination. This chapter focuses on common presentations in the examination and ultimately reflects common scenarios in clinical practice. Each scenario starts with a short introduction. In the examination there will be a similar introduction to read before you start the station. There is no allotted reading time, so read quickly but carefully!

For the history stations in the examination, you will only be expected to take a history – there is no requirement to examine the patient or to plan investigations. We have included a further discussion on investigations at the end of each section for reference.

1 Olfactory dysfunction
2 Nosebleeds in adults
3 Nosebleeds in children
4 Dry mouth
5 Lump in the throat
6 Hoarse voice
7 Catarrh and post-nasal drip
8 Tinnitus
9 Child with recurrent ear infections
10 Facial weakness
11 Septal perforation
12 Hearing loss in a child
13 Adult with itchy, painful ear
14 Adult with non-acute hearing loss
15 Adult with sudden hearing loss
16 Otalgia

1 Olfactory dysfunction

> 'A 70-year-old woman comes to your clinic reporting a change in her sense of smell for the last 2 months. Take a history from this patient.'

Olfactory dysfunction (OD) can arise from a variety of causes and has a surprisingly large impact on the patient's quality of life. Often it is the compromise of taste that the patient first notices.

OD can also lead to potentially dangerous situations, as the patient is unable to detect environmental hazards such as spoilt food or gas leaks. It is estimated that OD will affect 1% of the population under the age of 65 years and over 50% of the population older than 65 years.

General structure of the consultation

An understanding of the olfactory pathway will be your basis for structuring the consultation, as a problem at any level of the pathway can cause OD.

The olfactory pathway starts with sensory neurons in the nose. These detect odorants and transmit via the olfactory nerve (cranial nerve I) to the olfactory bulb located on top of the cribriform plate at the base of the frontal lobe. These subsequently transmit to the olfactory cortex. There is also an ancillary pathway transmitting somatosensory information such as temperature via the trigeminal nerve (cranial nerve V).

Some useful terms to begin with:
- anosmia – absence of smell function
- hyposmia – decreased sensitivity to odorants
- hyperosmia – increased sensitivity to odorants
- cacosmia – sensation of foul smells
- phantosmia – olfactory hallucination.

Structure your thinking around the possible causes of the OD. If you can work logically through these causes, you will not miss anything.

The OD can be:
- conductive – anything that stops odorant molecules getting to the receptors in the nose
- sensory – loss of receptor function
- neural – damage of peripheral and central olfactory pathways.

The most common causes you will be expected to know are:
- sinonasal disease

- postviral anosmia
- head trauma
- other, rarer causes (intracranial neoplasia; Addison's disease; Turner's, Cushing's or Kallmann's syndrome).

Specific questions

Start with an open question such as: 'I understand you are having some problems with your sense of smell. Perhaps you could tell me about these and how they are affecting you.'

This is a useful opening gambit, as it contextualises the patient's symptoms.

- When did you last have a normal sense of smell?
- Is it getting better or getting worse, or do you have bad episodes?
- Has there been any change since it started? Does your sense of smell fluctuate?
- Can you smell anything at all? Any unusual smells? (With this question you must be mindful that olfactory/auditory hallucinations can be a presenting feature of epilepsy. Patients often have preserved smell for noxious chemicals (e.g. strong perfume) through the trigeminal nerve.)
- Have you had any recent coughs or colds? (Postviral OD is the most common aetiology.)
- Have you had any trauma to your head? (Trauma to the skull base can disrupt olfactory neurons passing through the cribriform plate.)
- Do you have any problems with your nose normally? (Particularly, ask about nasal obstruction, discharge and its quality, epistaxis, allergies and polyps. Ascertain whether symptoms are uni- or bilateral.)
- Have you had headaches, fits, faints, loss of consciousness or vomiting? (These are signs of raised intracranial pressure (ICP) and need to be asked about to rule out intracranial neoplasia, a rare but important cause of OD.)
- Have you noticed anything else? (Use this opportunity to screen for associated features of nasal disease such as swellings in the head and neck, paraesthesia, facial pain – remember pain, epistaxis, obstruction and paraesthesia are 'red flag' symptoms that may suggest a malignant cause for the OD.)
- Have you had any surgery on the nose? (Patients with ongoing sinonasal disease will have often have had operative procedures. This correlates with OD as both cause and effect.)
- Have you noticed any change in your sense of taste? Does this interfere with eating?

Past medical history and general systems review

- Are you normally well in yourself? (Ask particularly about fevers, malaise, weight loss and systemic disease such as thyroid problems, diabetes and neurological conditions.)
- Have you noticed any changes in your memory? (Alzheimer's dementia and other neurodegenerative diseases have been associated with olfactory dysfunction.)
- Have you got children? (Explain that this may seem a strange question but Kallmann's syndrome (hypogonadotropic hypogonadism) can present with anosmia and impaired fertility.)

Close this part of the history by asking if they have anything else to tell you. This can be a useful time to screen for the patient's **I**deas, **C**oncerns and **E**xpectations.

Drug history

- Are you on any medication? (Ask particularly about antihypertensive and antihyperlipidaemic drugs, as these are known to be associated with OD.)
- Any allergies to medications?

Family history

- Do any conditions run in your family? (Ask about nasal polyposis, allergic rhinitis and cystic fibrosis that predispose to conductive OD.)

Social history

- What do you do for work? (Try to discover if there has been any exposure to toxic chemicals, e.g. nickel.)
- Do you smoke cigarettes?
- Do you have any pets or exposure to animals? (Allergic rhinitis can lead to OD.)

Further discussion: explanation and planning

Explain you would fully examine the patient's head and neck, obviously paying particular attention to the nose. Examine the nose in the standard fashion (*see* Chapter 2) paying attention to the nasal mucosa for signs of inflammation, deviation of the nasal septum and the presence of polyps. Explain you would perform nasal endoscopy with either the rigid or the flexible nasendoscope.

Explain that routinely other tests are only ordered as appropriate from the patient's history and examination findings and often no further investigation is helpful.

Blood tests can be used to rule out systemic disease (e.g. blood sugar, thyroid function tests).

If nasal pathology is detected on nasendoscopy (e.g. mucopus seen at the meatal orifices) then a computed tomography (CT) head with paranasal sinuses can be ordered to delineate the degree of sinonasal disease, in planning for possible operative intervention.

CT imaging is also required if the patient presents with a constellation of 'red flag' symptoms as already detailed.

If no nasal pathology is detected then magnetic resonance imaging (MRI) of the head/olfactory pathway can be used to rule out uncommon tumours such a meningiomas and aesthesioblastomas.

Qualitative assessment of smell can be performed using the University of Pennsylvania Smell Identification Test (rarely used in clinical practice).

Discuss treatment options depending on results of the investigations (e.g. sinosnasal disease, tumours).

If sensorineural anosmia (most often of postviral origin) is diagnosed, explain that there are no specific treatments. Spontaneous recovery is sometimes possible, although the defect is permanent in the majority of cases.

Patient reassurance and education is important, warning specifically about the risk of gas leaks and contaminated food.

2 Nosebleeds in adults

'A 45-year-old man attends your outpatient clinic reporting repeated nose-bleeds over the last few months.'

Although epistaxis is a common occurrence in all age groups, typically it has a bimodal distribution presenting in children and the elderly. The nose has a rich blood supply from both the internal (anterior and posterior ethmoid arteries) and external carotid arteries (facial and internal maxillary arteries). Bleeding is classically described as originating from the anterior or posterior septum, although the distinction between these is somewhat arbitrary. Anterior bleeds are most often from Little's area (an area where the internal and external carotid arteries anastomose), whereas posterior bleeds are more often from the sphenopalatine artery or are of venous origin.

General structure of the consultation

Most cases will not have a singular cause but will be the result of a number of concomitant factors such as nasal trauma, rhinitis, hypertension and anticoagulation. These risk factors tend to increase with age, hence the increasing prevalence in the elderly population. It is important to differentiate these cases from those that may have a more sinister cause, such as intranasal malignancy.

Specific questions

- How long have you been having nosebleeds?
- How often do they occur?
- When you have a nosebleed, how long does it last?
- How much blood do you lose? (Measures such as an egg cup, teaspoon, etc., can be useful to quantify amounts.)
- Does it come from one side or both sides?
- Does blood come into the mouth? (This may be indicative of posterior bleeds.)
- What do you do to stop the bleeding? (This question can also ascertain whether they have an understanding of first aid.)
- Have you required hospital treatment to stop the bleeding in the past?
- Do you have any associated nasal symptoms? (Ask particularly about nasal obstruction, pain, discharge, crusting, paraesthesia, lymphadenopathy in the head and neck. These are 'red flag' symptoms for intranasal malignancy.)
- Have you had any trauma to the nose? (Particularly ask about nasal picking.)

* Any exposure to animals/pollen? (Allergens are a common cause of epistaxis, by causing inflammation and hyperaemia of the nasal mucosa.)
* Ask about how the condition is affecting the patient, e.g interfering with social function and so forth. This is a useful place to screen for any 'hidden agendas'.

Past medical history and general systems review
* Ask about hypertension, heart disease, bleeding diatheses and liver disease. These are all known bleeding-risk factors.

Drug history
* Do you take any blood-thinning tablets? (Particularly, warfarin, aspirin and clopidogrel.)
* Do you use intranasal oxygen? (This predisposes to epistaxis by drying the nasal mucosa.)
* Ask sensitively about intranasal drug use, e.g. cocaine.
* Any allergies to medications?

Family history
* Do any blood clotting disorders run in your family? (Hereditary coagulopathies predispose to epistaxis.)

Social history
* Do you smoke or drink alcohol?

Further discussion: explanation and planning
Explain you would examine the patient's head and neck, paying particular attention to the nose and nasal septum.

Often with anterior bleeding points you can visualise a septal vessel that can be cauterised. A week of intranasal antibiotic such as Naseptin cream can then be prescribed.

If there is no obvious bleeding point to visualise on anterior rhinoscopy, you would perform rigid endoscopy.

Blood tests are rarely necessary. However, in cases of severe blood loss with suspected anaemia, or in cases where there is the suspicion of an underlying coagulopathy, a full blood count (FBC) and clotting profile should be ordered.

With patients on warfarin the international normalised ratio (INR) should be checked (their 'yellow book' should document the normal range for their INR).

Patients with 'red flag' symptoms for neoplasia should undergo CT examination of the head and paranasal sinuses.

If the patient does not have a working knowledge of first aid measures then these should be explained. For example, place the head forwards and pinch the soft part of the nose, and ice on the back of the neck can also be tried.

Explain to the patient that any bleeds that do not stop with first aid require them to come in to hospital. Initially it is very likely that nasal cautery will be attempted; severe bleeding may require recourse to nasal packing and a stay as an inpatient.

In recurrent nosebleeds, refractory to more conservative management, surgical ligation of the bleeding vessel, e.g. sphenopalatine artery ligation or radiological embolisation, is possible.

3 Nosebleeds in children

> 'A 10-year-old girl comes to clinic with her mother who tells you the child has been having two or three nosebleeds a week for the last year.'

Nosebleeds are a common complaint in children. The vast majority are not serious; however, they are often a source of serious parental concern and a source of social embarrassment for the child. As with adult epistaxis, bleeds can be classified on their site of origin: either anterior or posterior. Anterior bleeds from Kiesselbach's plexus/Little's area (where anterior and posterior ethmoid and sphenopalatine/internal maxillary arteries anastomose) are the most common. In older children most epistaxes result from nasal trauma or nasal picking; however, nasal foreign bodies are also common.

General structure of the consultation

This is a similar structure to the history for nosebleeds in adults (*see* Section 2), with some specific additions. You will be faced with an actor playing the parent; there will never be children in the examination. Think about the possible causes of a nosebleed in a child to help structure your approach to this station.

Causes include:
- nasal picking
- allergies
- infection
- trauma
- very rarely, neoplasia.

Specific questions

- How long has she been having nosebleeds?
- How often do they occur?
- How long do they last?
- How much blood does she lose? (Refer to familiar quantities such as an egg cup to help the mother here.)
- Does it come from one side or from both sides?
- Does it come into the mouth?
- What do you do to stop the bleeding?
- Has she had any treatment in the past?
- Any associated nasal symptoms? (Ask particularly about nasal obstruction, pain, discharge, crusting, paraesthesias, and swellings in the head and neck. These are 'red flag' symptoms for intranasal malignancy.)

◆ Has she had any trauma to the nose? (Particularly ask about nasal picking.)

◆ What is the impact on her life? (Ask about problems at school – recurrent nosebleeds can be socially isolating.)

◆ Does she have any exposure to animals/pollen? (Allergens are a common cause of epistaxis, by causing inflammation and hyperaemia of the nasal mucosa.)

◆ Try to elucidate the mother's **I**deas, **C**oncerns and **E**xpectations, as it is very likely she will be anxious about serious underlying pathology.

Past medical history and general systems review

◆ Is she otherwise well? (Ask about weight and development, fevers and malaise. These are useful questions for ruling out systemic disease.)

◆ Has she had any unexpected bruising or bleeding from other sites? (Many haematological disorders can present with epistaxis, e.g. childhood leukaemias.)

Drug history

◆ Is she on any medications?

◆ Any allergies to medications?

Family history

◆ Any conditions run in the family?

Social history

◆ Does she have any siblings? If so, similar problems?

◆ Any smoking in the household? (This predisposes to epistaxis by irritating the nasal mucosa.)

Further discussion: explanation and planning

Explain you would examine the child's head and neck, paying particular attention to the nose and nasal septum. The first-line treatment would be a 10-day course of Naseptin. Cautery is a second-line therapy, as it is often difficult in children. If you are unable to perform a satisfactory examination and the child is having severe symptoms, then suggest an examination under anaesthetic may be appropriate.

Rigid endoscopy is surprisingly well tolerated by children and should be performed if there is no initially obvious cause for the bleeding.

Explain blood tests are not usually required but may be appropriate in heavy recurrent bleeds or when there is suspicion of an underlying haematological condition.

In exceptional cases, MRI of the head may be appropriate to rule out neoplasia.

Reassure appropriately, as most children will grow out of nosebleeds. Often a short course of intranasal antibiotic such as Naseptin is all that is needed.

Educate the parent about first aid techniques if they are not familiar with them.

4 Dry mouth

'A 70-year-old man complains of a dry mouth for the last 6 months.'

Saliva is produced from three pairs of major salivary glands (parotid, submandibular and sublingual) and multiple minor salivary glands throughout the mouth. Saliva is primarily water, with small quantities of dissolved mucus, enzymes and electrolytes. The main role of saliva is to aid the production of a moistened food bolus that can be swallowed. The presence of salivary enzymes amylase and lipase also play an initial role in digestion. The normal adult produces and subsequently swallows approximately 1 L of saliva every day.

Salivation is under control of the autonomic nervous system. The decreased production of saliva is a normal physiological part of the 'fight-or-flight response' (sympathetic overdrive). However, a persistent dry mouth can become a source of morbidity, making chewing, eating and talking difficult.

General structure of the consultation

The correct medical term for a dry mouth is xerostomia, defined as the real or apparent sensation of hyposalivation.

It is important to think about possible causes for the dry mouth to help structure your thinking when approaching this station. Disruption to any part of the pathway from the brain to the salivary gland can cause underproduction of saliva. Hence, you should consider sensory (disruption to taste sensation can cause hyposalivation), neural (damage to any part of the neural pathway, including cranial nerves VII, IX and V) and secretomotor dysfunction (direct damage to the salivary glands).

Common causes include:

- Medication side effects – any drug with effects on the autonomic nervous system can cause xerostomia. Antihypertensives and antidepressants are particularly well known in this regard.
- Mouth breathing – this may be due to nasal blockage, e.g from adenoidal hypertrophy.
- Systemic disease – autoimmune disease such as Sjögren's syndrome must be ruled out. Other systemic disease such as human immunodeficiency virus (HIV), diabetes and Parkinson's disease can also cause dry mouth.
- Radiation therapy – the salivary glands, particularly the parotid glands, are often in the radiation field during treatment of head and neck cancer. A number of new developments including intensity-modulated radiotherapy

have been developed to minimise collateral damage to healthy salivary tissue.

◈ Pseudoxerostomia, rarely as a manifestation of psychiatric disease.

Specific questions

◈ How long has your mouth been dry?

◈ Is it dry all the time or in episodes?

◈ Is it dry when you are eating? Does the sensation of dryness stop you eating?

◈ Any problems with your sense of taste and smell?

◈ Do you have any problems swallowing? (Swallowing problems are a 'red flag' and should heighten your awareness of underlying malignancy.)

◈ Do you feel that you don't have enough saliva in your mouth?

◈ Do you sleep well? Do you snore? (Disturbed sleep and snoring predispose to loss of hydration of the oral mucosa.)

◈ Do you breathe through your nose or mouth? (Nasal obstruction can predispose to mouth breathing and hence dryness of the oral mucosa.)

◈ Any bad breath? Any problems with your teeth or infections of the mouth? (The loss of saliva increases the growth of pathogenic oral microflora and hence the risk of cavities and intra-oral infection.)

◈ Screen for the patient's Ideas, Concerns and Expectations.

Past medical history and general systems review

◈ Are you usually well? (Ask specifically about diabetes, autoimmune disease and neurological disease.)

◈ Any recent coughs or colds?

◈ Have you noticed any dryness of the eyes, rash, arthritis, or Raynaud's phenomenon? (These are the symptoms of Sjögren's syndrome.)

◈ Have you had any cancers of the head and neck region? (Ask specifically about radiation exposure.)

Drug history

◈ Are you on any medications? (This is an extremely common cause of a dry mouth and a number of different classes of medication have xerostomia listed as a side effect.)

◈ Any allergies to medications?

Family history

◈ Does anyone in your family suffer from a similar problem? (Ask specifically about a history of autoimmune disease.)

Social history

◆ Do you smoke or drink alcohol?

◆ Ask sensitively about risk factors for HIV exposure (sexual history, intravenous drug use).

◆ What do you do for work? (Ask about voice abuse, e.g. teachers, singers – a rare but possible cause of a dry mouth.)

Further discussion: explanation and planning

Explain you would examine the patient's head and neck fully, paying particular attention to the mouth and salivary glands.

Other investigations will depend on the history and examination findings.

Plan blood glucose levels to rule out diabetes.

Plan FBC, urea and electrolytes (U+Es), liver function tests, immunological tests including rheumatoid factor, SS-A, SS-B (Sjögren's syndrome A- and B-antibodies) if autoimmune disease is suspected

Sialometry can be used to quantify saliva production, but this is very rarely used outside of a research setting.

Plan biopsy of a lip minor salivary gland for histology to diagnose primary Sjögren's syndrome.

Plan imaging studies such as magnetic resonance sialography or more commonly ultrasound scan (USS) of the major salivary glands.

Treatment depends on the cause, e.g. stringent glucose control in diabetes, medication rationalisation, stopping smoking or referral to rheumatology service if autoimmune condition is diagnosed.

Symptom management consists of frequent oral lubrication with fluids, artificial saliva, sialogogues (e.g. pilocarpine) and the use of chewing gum to stimulate saliva production.

5 Lump in the throat

'A 55-year-old lawyer presents to your outpatient clinic with a feeling of something in her throat for the last 4 months.'

General structure of the consultation
The feeling of something in the throat (FOSIT) has diverse causative factors. Generally these can be split into benign and malignant. The majority of cases will be idiopathic (globus pharyngeus) in origin, with reassurance and education being the mainstay of treatment. It is crucial to rule out malignant disease. However, malignancy rarely presents solely with FOSIT. Therefore, the history is vital in diagnosis of the underlying problem. Another point to mention is that in the examination setting, these patients often have a 'hidden agenda' or very specific worries about what might be causing their symptoms. There will be marks for finding out the cause of their anxiety.

Specific questions
◆ Ask the patient to describe in her own words exactly the sensation she is getting. (Sensations range from a feeling of phlegm running down or sticking at the back of the throat to foreign body sensation with concomitant dysphagia.)
◆ How long have you had this sensation?
◆ Is it getting better or worse? (Globus pharyngeus is by and large a non-progressive condition.)
◆ Does it come in episodes or is it present all the time?
◆ Is it better when eating? Has it ever interfered with eating? (Classically globus sensation goes away when swallowing, but this is not always the case.)
◆ Do you have any pain or trouble swallowing? (This is an important question, as any dysphagia or odynophagia should prompt further questioning and investigation. Important features include the time course, progression, worsening with solids or liquid (worse with liquids implies neurological disease) and regurgitation (pharyngeal pouch).)
◆ Any changes in your voice? (Voice change is a 'red flag' symptom for upper aerodigestive tract neoplasia (*see* Section 6, Hoarse voice).)
◆ Any new lumps in the head or neck? (Lymphadenopathy is an important feature of both infection and malignancy.)
◆ Do you suffer from heartburn or regurgitation?

◆ Any pain in your ears? (Referred otalgia is a 'red flag' symptom for neoplasia of the head and neck (*see* Section 16, Otalgia).)

Past medical history and general systems review

◆ How have you been in yourself lately? (Screen for weight loss, fevers, malaise, chest symptoms such as haemoptysis and shortness of breath.)
◆ Ask about systemic illnesses and particularly screen for depression and psychiatric problems, including other healthcare-seeking behaviour or medically unexplained symptoms.

Drug history

◆ Do you take any medications?
◆ Any allergies to medications?

Social history

◆ Do you smoke or drink alcohol?
◆ What do you do for work?
◆ Ask about general anxiety levels and worries. It is important to try to explore the patient's **I**deas, **C**oncerns and **E**xpectations, as frequently these patients have a 'hidden agenda'.

Further discussion: explanation and planning

Explain you would perform a thorough examination of the neck, including the neck lymph nodes and thyroid gland.

Explain you would perform flexible nasendoscopy to rule out any lesions of the upper aerodigestive tract.

If no abnormalities have been found and the history is suggestive of globus pharyngeus, then the patient can be reassured. Often a reassurance that there is no abnormality detected is all that the patient needs. In the clinical setting it can be useful to allow the patient to see their own aerodigestive tract using the flexible nasendoscope and video stack.

In patients who still remain anxious, it is important for them to remove focus from the sensation. They should be encouraged to break the swallow-sensation cycle where dry swallowing worsens the sensation rather than eases it.

If the history and examination prove normal, further investigation such as barium swallows is generally not required. This is particulary true in younger non-smokers.

Laryngopharyngeal reflux (LPR) has been implicated in globus sensation;

however, the efficacy of proton-pump inhibitors (PPIs) is still debated. The role of cognitive behavioural therapy (CBT) is also equivocal.

If more worrisome symptoms are revealed in the history, such as weight loss, constant and progressive dysphagia or pain (e.g. referred otalgia or odynophagia), then further investigation will be required. The first-line investigation is a barium swallow and rigid endoscopy with or without biopsies. Many head and neck surgeons will perform panendoscopy as a first-line treatment in any patient they feel is at high risk of malignancy.

6 Hoarse voice

> 'A 64-year-old ex-publican presents to the outpatients clinic with a 4-month history of a hoarse voice.'

The production of the human voice can be divided into three parts:
1 production of airflow from the lungs
2 vibration of the vocal folds
3 articulation from the soft palate and tongue.

A dysphonia is a disorder of the ability to produce normal vocal sounds and it can result from impairment at any part of the vocal tract.

General structure of the consultation

This is a common presentation in outpatients and, as ever, there is a multiplicity of causes, both functional and organic. It is of the utmost importance to differentiate those of a benign and those of a malignant nature. The most common dysphonic voice is a hoarse voice. The most common reason for hoarseness is the interruption of normal vocal fold vibration.

The most common causes that you will be expected to know for the examination are:

- laryngitis – this can be either infective (viral/bacterial) or caused by local irritants such as smoking or LPR)
- voice abuse – this is often related to the patient's occupation or hobby (e.g. teachers, singers)
- local vocal cord disease (e.g. cysts, nodules, Reinke's oedema)
- neoplasia – particularly squamous cell carcinomas (SCCs) of the larynx
- endocrine (diabetes, hypothyroidism)
- haematological (leukaemia, lymphoma, amyloidosis).

Specific questions

Start with an open question asking the patient to explain what changes they have noticed in their voice. This gives you a good opportunity to objectively assess the patient's voice.

- How long have the changes been happening for?
- Did they happen gradually or did they have a sudden onset? (Neoplasia tends to cause a gradually increasing hoarseness.)
- Is your voice getting better or worse?
- Does your voice have times when it is normal or is it always hoarse?

◆ Anything bring this on? For example, sustained vocal use or after periods of heavy smoking.

◆ Do you ever lose your voice completely?

◆ Have you had any recent coughs or colds? (This may be indicative of an infective laryngitis.)

◆ Do you clear your throat a lot?

◆ Do you have the feeling of catarrh or sticking phlegm?

◆ Do you cough a lot? Is it worse when lying down?

◆ Do you get symptoms of acid reflux (gastro-oesophageal reflux)? (This may overlap with LPR and predispose to pepsin-induced changes to the vocal folds.)

◆ Do you have a sensation of something in your throat?

◆ Any problems swallowing? (Any problem swallowing or FOSIT should prompt further investigation, as this is a common presentation of upper aerodigestive tract tumours (*see* Section 5, Lump in the throat).)

◆ Any pain in the throat or ears? (This can be primary or referred.)

◆ Any heartburn or chest pain?

◆ Any shortness of breath or haemoptysis? (This is important, as chest disease may manifest as dysphonia due to inadequate airflow production.)

◆ Any new lumps in the head or neck? (Lymphadenopathy can result from local disease but it can also result from lung cancer. Thyroid enlargement can also be a causative factor.)

◆ Screen for the patient's **I**deas, **C**oncerns and **E**xpectations.

Past medical history and general systems review

◆ Are you generally a well person? (Ask specifically about weight loss, fever and malaise as signs of systemic disease.)

◆ Ask specifically about diabetes, thyroid disease and neurological conditions. These can present as voice changes, although this is rarely the only symptom.

◆ Ask specifically about chest and heart disease, as both can cause hoarseness. Ask about previous thoracic surgery, a known risk factor for recurrent laryngeal nerve damage.

◆ Have you had any surgery? (Any procedure under general anaesthetic may give rise to the traumatic effects of intubation.)

Drug history

◆ Are you on any medications?

◆ Any allergies to medications?

Family history

◈ Do any conditions run in the family?

Social history

◈ Do you smoke or drink alcohol?

◈ What do you do for work? (Ask about voice abuse, e.g. teachers, singers.)

Further discussion: explanation and planning

Explain you would fully examine the head and neck and perform flexible nasendoscopy (FNE), paying particular attention to the larynx.

You should ask the patient to read a standard paragraph or to count to 10. The voice can then be graded on the GRBAS (grade, roughness, breathiness, asthenia, strain) scale, with each characteristic given a grading between 1 and 4 (where 4 is a severe disturbance).

If the history and examination point to a functional cause, reassurance and education is important. It is advisable for the patient to avoid situations that strain the voice. A period of voice rest can be advised. General smoking and drinking advice should be given.

Most patients will get better with these lifestyle changes; however, referral to a voice therapist or specialist voice clinic is appropriate for chronic cases.

In patients describing acid reflux symptoms, LPR may account for their dysphonia. The role of LPR is poorly understood. However, in patients with reflux symptoms, a trial of PPIs and alginate solutions (which also stop pepsin and bile acid regurgitation by forming a physical barrier) is a reasonable course of action.

Surgery is appropriate for organic lesions such as polyps and for medialisation of paralysed cords. For idiopathic vocal cord palsies it is normal practice to wait at least 1 year to allow spontaneous return of normal voice.

Patients at high risk of malignancy or with lesions visible with FNE should proceed to microlaryngoscopy positive/negative biopsies under general anaesthetic. These patients should have an initial chest X-ray (CXR) and CT of the neck and chest.

Treatment of malignant disease will be as part of a multidisciplinary team and it will involve surgery, radiotherapy or both.

7 Catarrh and post-nasal drip

'A 47-year-old female shopworker reports the feeling of mucus running down the back of her throat. She tells you that her throat has been itchy for many years.'

Catarrh is a non-specific term used by patients for a number of different symptom patterns. These range from a productive cough to nasal obstruction. The wide variety of symptoms requires careful history taking, as the causative factors are wide-ranging. Typically, catarrh is defined as inflammation of the mucous membranes of the upper airways causing an excess of mucus. Patients often describe a feeling of mucus 'running down' their throat. In some patients, catarrh persists due to underlying organic disease such as allergies or abnormalities like nasal polyps. However, it is common that no underlying abnormality can be detected; where this is the case, education and reassurance is the mainstay of treatment.

General structure of the consultation

This is often a difficult consultation and a bit of manoeuvring is required to align the patient's demands with what you can deliver as a clinician. It is important to differentiate patients who are actually overproducing mucus from those who only have the sensation that they are. It can be helpful to ask the patient to rank their symptoms in order of severity. It is common that patients present with a number of different chronic symptoms that they attribute to mucus overproduction, e.g. nausea, headaches and tiredness.

Specific questions

- Ask them to describe the symptoms they are experiencing.
- How long have you had these symptoms?
- Are you getting better or worse?
- Do you get worse at a particular time?
- Do you have a cough?
- Any production of mucus with the cough? (Ask about the quality of the mucus – its colour, its consistency and the presence of blood. Many patients feel an inability to shift mucus from their chests (failed expectoration) and this can be a source of great anxiety and annoyance.)
- Do you have a blocked nose?
- Any nasal discharge, sinus pain or anosmia? (These may indicate underlying sinusitis, which can be diagnosed on the presence of two major factors or

one major and two minor factors, in addition to evidence of inflamed sinus mucosa or pus visualised with nasendoscopy. Major factors are facial pain, nasal obstruction, nasal discharge, anosmia and fever. Minor factors are headache, halitosis, fatigue, dental pain and cough.)
- Do you have any allergies? (Sneezing fits and epiphora are symptoms of allergic rhinitis.)
- Do you have any facial pain? (The presence of pain may indicate underlying infection or sinusitis.)
- Screen for the patient's **I**deas, **C**oncerns and **E**xpectations.

Past medical history and general systems review
- Ask about weight loss, malaise, fevers.
- Ask about any other systemic disease that can predispose to immune compromise and subsequent infection, e.g. diabetes, HIV.

Drug history
- Are you on any medications?
- Any allergies to medications?

Family history
- Do any conditions run in the family?

Social history
- Do you smoke or drink alcohol?
- What do you do for work?

Further discussion: explanation and planning
Explain that you will examine the nose and post-nasal space (PNS) with anterior rhinoscopy and FNE/rigid endoscopy.

Plan treatment of chronic rhinosinusitis or allergies as appropriate.

If no organic cause found, reassurance and learning to cope with symptoms is the key management strategy. Investigations should not be used to reassure patients.

Nasal steroids may be of benefit. Patients often find saline nasal rinses useful.

8 Tinnitus

'A 70-year-old man comes to your outpatient clinic reporting a 10-year history of ringing in his ears, which he particularly notices when he is trying to sleep.'

Tinnitus is perception of sound within the ear in the absence of any external sound. It is a very common complaint and it typically takes the form of a ringing noise. It is reported that one in three of the adult population have some tinnitus experience.

Tinnitus can be sensed in one or both ears or more non-specifically 'inside the head'. Broadly, tinnitus can be classified as objective (a sound perceived by the clinician, e.g. a bruit) or subjective (a sound only perceived by the patient). Tinnitus is subjective in the vast majority of cases.

General structure of the consultation

In clinical practice, most often the only coincident pathology is sensorineural hearing loss (SNHL). However, it is important to differentiate these cases from cases caused by more sinister pathologies such as vestibular schwannoma or other specific otological diseases like Ménière's syndrome.

The pathogenesis of tinnitus is far from understood. A number of models have been used to explain some of the underlying complexities. For example, one model defines an 'ignition site' caused by perturbation anywhere in the auditory system and a 'promotion site' where the initial signal is enhanced and occurring in the central auditory system. This is then overlaid with anxiety/psychosomatic effects.

Important causes include:
- Otological – noise trauma, ear infection, otitis media, wax impaction, presbycusis/SNHL, Ménière's syndrome, vestibular schwannoma, other skull base tumours (e.g. glomus tympanicum).
- Medications, e.g. aspirin (not at therapeutic dose), non-steroidal anti-inflammatory drugs, ototoxic antibiotics, e.g. gentamicin, cisplatin (many other drugs list tinnitus as a side effect; however, there is scant evidence for causation for most).
- Systemic disease – thyroid disease, vitamin B_{12} deficiency, anaemia.
- Psychiatric disease – anxiety, depression.

Specific questions
- Ask them to describe the symptoms they are getting.

◈ How long have you experienced this?

◈ Is it intermittent or is it always there?

◈ How loud is it?

◈ Is it on one side or both sides? (Unilateral tinnitus requires the possibility of a skull base lesion to be ruled out by intracranial imaging.)

◈ Is the symptom worse with noise or worse in silence?

◈ What is the character of the noise? (This can often be classified as pulsatile, ringing or clicking.)

◈ What is your hearing like? (Tinnitus is often associated with hearing loss.)

◈ Are you ever troubled by very loud sounds? (Hyperacusis may indicate recruitment with hearing loss.)

◈ Do you have any pain in the ears?

◈ Any discharge?

◈ Any fullness?

◈ Any vertigo or sense of imbalance? (A combination of aural fullness, hearing loss, tinnitus and vertigo may suggest the possibility of vestibular schwannoma or Ménière's syndrome.)

◈ Does it stop you sleeping? (Sleep disturbance is often reported that may exacerbate underlying anxiety and propagate the vicious cycle.)

◈ How is it affecting your life? Screen for signs of depression and anxiety and the patient's **I**deas, **C**oncerns and **E**xpectations. You should specifically explore the patient's fears of having a brain tumour. This is a common concern in the examination and in clinical practice.

Drug history

◈ Are you on any medications? (A number of drugs have been associated with tinnitus including over-the-counter herbal supplements. Aspirin, antimalarials, diuretics, ototoxic antibiotics and benzodiazepines are known to be associated with SNHL and hence tinnitus.)

◈ Any allergies to medications?

Family history

◈ Do any conditions run in the family?

Social history

◈ Do you smoke or drink alcohol?

◈ What do you do for work?

Further discussion: explanation and planning

Explain you would perform a full head and neck examination.

Otoscopy to check for obvious otological pathology and middle ear pathology including glomus tumours (pulsatile tinnitus); in this case, auscultation of the ear for a bruit should be performed.

Audiometry is required to document the baseline hearing level.

Plan examination of fundi for signs of raised ICP.

Formal vestibular function tests are occasionally required if there is a history of vestibular dysfunction.

Cranial nerve examination – skull base lesions can impinge on cranial nerves as they enlarge, producing focal neurological signs.

Plan MRI of the head (with gadolinium contrast if normal renal function) if a tumour is suspected, e.g. from unilateral tinnitus, signs of raised ICP.

Without specific otological disease, surgery is not recommended (previous cochlear destruction/nerve sectioning are of limited effectiveness and offer serious risk to the patient).

Management of otological disease such as chronic suppurative otitis media (CSOM) or otosclerosis has variable outcomes on tinititus.

If there is no organic pathology, the treatment is conservative: reassurance, counselling, CBT, tinnitus retraining therapy, white noise generators for masking, hearing aids for SNHL.

There is no role for medication: although a number of therapies have been tried over the years, the evidence for any particular treatment is sparse.

Lidocaine has been shown to be effective in some research cases when given intravenously; the search for an orally active derivative continues.

There are a number of active clinical trials looking for pharmacological agents, e.g. N-methyl-D-aspartic acid antagonists.

9 Child with recurrent ear infections

'A 4-year-old girl attends your ear, nose and throat (ENT) clinic with a history of recurrent "ear infections".'

General structure of the consultation

Here it is important to find out what type of infection the child is getting. In the examination setting there will never be a child at the station; instead, your questioning will be directed to the parent. Acute otitis media (AOM) is the most common presentation in this age group. However, this needs to be differentiated from other infections (e.g. otitis externa (OE), although this is rare in childhood).

AOM is an inflammation of the middle ear manifesting with both local and systemic symptoms. Common symptoms include otalgia, discharge, fever, ear tugging, nausea and decreased appetite.

The causative agent is often viral (respiratory syncytial virus, adenovirus) but it can also be bacterial (*Streptococcus pneumoniae*, *Haemophilus influenzae*). There is increasing evidence that the microbiology of AOM is changing with the introduction of the polyvalent pneumococcal vaccine.

AOM is an extremely common condition, with almost all children having at least one episode. Approximately 10% of children experience four or more episodes in a year. AOM has a negative impact on the quality of life of both the child and the parents. It is important to remember AOM has potentially serious sequelae, including intracranial abscess and meningitis.

Specific questions

- What symptoms is she getting? (Ask specifically about ear tugging, ear discharge, feeding patterns, fevers and lethargy.)
- How long has she been getting episodes?
- How frequent are the episodes?
- How long do the episodes last?
- Has she received antibiotics in the past?
- Has she been unwell recently? (Ask specifically about coughs, colds and rhinorrhea. AOM is often preceded by upper respiratory tract infections (URTIs). Before 6 months there is passive immunity from transplacental IgG. In older children, recurrent cases may need investigation for immunocompromise, particularly if there are other recurrent infections, e.g. URTI.)

◆ How is her hearing and speech and language development? (It can be helpful to make a comparison with any other children in the family or the child's peer group at school.)

◆ How are they managing at school? Have the teachers noticed anything?

◆ Does the child snore at night? (Ask about signs of sleep apnoea or nasal obstruction that can predispose to AOM and otitis media with effusion (OME).)

Past medical history and general systems review

◆ Is she normally well in herself?

◆ Has she had her routine immunisations? (A new pneumococcal vaccine is currently under investigation for preventing AOM.)

◆ Has she had any other infections? (Any history of other infections may be suggestive of immunocompromise.)

◆ Was she a full-term baby? (Ask about the foetal and neonatal history.)

Drug history

◆ Is she on any medications?

◆ Any allergies to medications?

Family history

◆ Do any conditions run in the family?

Social history

◆ Is there any smoking in the household? (An important environmental risk factor.)

◆ Any siblings of the child affected similarly?

Further discussion: explanation and planning

Explain you would perform a full examination of the child's head and neck, centring on the ears and the mouth (for cleft palate) and nose (for obstruction).

An irritable, clinically unwell child with the classic bulging, red tympanic membrane (TM) on otoscopy is diagnostic of AOM.

Often the TM has perforated and the canal is filled with pus. Middle ear pus can be distinguished from OE by its quality and pulsatility (due to middle ear vasculature).

Perform age-appropriate hearing tests.

The general body of evidence is that AOM should be treated with antibiotics in children less than 18 months old. In older children, a watchful waiting period of 48–72 hours is reasonable. Failure to progress after this time is indication for antibiotics (at the expense of increased risk of side effects).

Recurrent AOM can be treated with low-dose daily amoxicillin. As appropriate, it may be necessary to screen for immunocompromise with levels of serum immunoglobulins.

Myringotomy and grommet insertion is a reasonable treatment for children with recurrent disease, particularly if there are frequent infections with perforations and discharge.

10 Facial weakness

'A 40-year-old man is referred to your clinic with a history of a unilateral facial weakness for the last 2 days.'

The facial nerve (cranial nerve VII) is derived from the second branchial arch and contains motor, sensory and parasympathetic fibres. The facial motor nucleus is in the pons.

The motor branch supplies the muscles of facial expression: buccinators, stylohyoid, stapedius, posterior belly of digastrics and platysma. The sensory branch carries taste via the chorda tympani.

The parasympathetic component supplies the secretomotor function for the submandibular/sublingual salivary glands and nasal, lacrimal and palatine mucosal glands.

The nerve is classically divided into four subsections: a cerebellopontine, internal acoustic meatus, intratemporal and an extratemporal division.

Facial nerve weakness is classified on the House–Brackmann classification of facial nerve palsy (I for normal to VI for no movement).

General structure of the consultation

When structuring this consultation it is important to keep mindful of the anatomy of the nerve. This will help you give a logical format and ensure that possible causes are not forgotten. Facial weakness can occur with impairment at any part of the neuromuscular tract.

The most common causes of facial weakness are:
- Bell's palsy (idiopathic facial nerve palsy)
- Ramsay Hunt syndrome (herpes zoster oticus)
- neoplasia, e.g. parotid malignancy
- trauma, e.g. birth trauma or skull base fracture
- infection, e.g. AOM/CSOM or Lyme disease
- congenital
- central nervous system dysfunction, e.g. stroke.

Although the differential diagnosis of a facial nerve weakness is broad, the history and examination significantly aid in diagnosis.

Specific questions
- When did the weakness start?
- What did you first notice?

◈ Is it just one side or have you noticed changes to the other side?

◈ Did it come on suddenly or has it been coming on gradually? (The time course is not always instructive, as all causes can progress at similar rates. However, in cases that are not improving after 6 weeks, further investigation to rule out neoplasia should be undertaken.)

◈ Have you had any recent coughs or colds? (Postviral facial palsy is a common cause.)

◈ Have you had any changes to your ears? (Ask specifically about otalgia, vesicles, hearing loss, vertigo, tinnitus and discharge. These are specific questions for associated otological disease. Possibilities that should be considered include AOM with a dehiscent facial nerve, malignant OE, cholesteatoma and skull base neoplasia.)

◈ Any surgery to the ears?

◈ Have you had any trauma to your head lately? (Temporal bone fractures can compromise the nerve.)

◈ Have you been at depth or to high altitude recently? (Patients with a dehiscent facial nerve canal can present with facial baroparesis, which tends to be a self-resolving neuropraxia.)

◈ Have you noticed any other weaknesses or sensory disturbances in the rest of the body? (Other CNS pathology, e.g. multiple sclerosis or stroke, should always be considered.)

Past medical history and general systems review

◈ Do you have any other conditions? (Ask specifically about hypertension and diabetes.)

◈ Have you ever had a cancer or tumour diagnosed? (Metastatic disease from other head and neck primary sites is possible.)

◈ Any family history of similar occurrences? (Melkersson–Rosenthal syndrome (lip oedema, recurrent facial weakness and fissuring of the tongue) can be hereditary.)

Drug history

◈ Are you on any medications?

◈ Any allergies to medications?

Family history

◈ Do any conditions run in the family?

Social history

◆ Do you smoke or drink alcohol?

◆ What do you do for work?

◆ Have you been travelling recently? (For example, to areas where Lyme disease is endemic.)

Further discussion: explanation and planning

Explain you would perform a full examination of the facial nerve and grade the weakness (e.g. using the House–Brackmann scale).

The weakness should be classified into upper motor neuron (UMN) or lower motor neuron (LMN) lesion. Because of bicortical representation there is forehead sparing in a UMN lesion, e.g. with a cerebral vascular accident. With an LMN palsy, e.g. Bell's palsy, there will be weakness in all divisions of the face.

Plan full examination of the ipsilateral ear and mastoid.

Plan full cranial nerve examination; check cranial nerve V in particular, as paraesthesia or pain in this distribution can be a sign of acoustic neuroma – Hitselberger's sign.

Plan flexible nasendoscopy, to rule out a nasopharyngeal cancer. These can involve any of the cranial nerves. By this stage in progression it is very likely that other, lower cranial nerves will also be compromised.

Plan full examination of the parotid gland to rule out a parotid tumour. A parotid mass with facial nerve palsy is suggestive of malignancy, e.g. mucoepidermoid, adenoid cystic subtypes.

Pure-tone audiometry (PTA) should be performed to document the baseline hearing level.

Treatment: first, educate about eye protection. This is particularly important at night, as corneal drying can result in corneal ulceration and, ultimately, blindness.

If an obvious cause is found such as parotid mass then manage this appropriately, e.g. perform fine needle aspiration (FNA) for histology.

Blood tests, e.g. Lyme disease serology, should only be performed if indicated from the history.

In the absence of an obvious diagnosis it is appropriate to make an initial diagnosis of Bell's palsy. A 7- to 10-day reducing dose of corticosteroid improves prognosis. Antivirals have not been shown to improve recovery but are still used by many clinicians.

Ramsay Hunt syndrome (varicella zoster infection manifesting as facial weakness and otic vesicles) is routinely treated with a course of aciclovir and reducing corticosteroids.

The patient should be followed up in 3–4 weeks. Lack of recovery may indicate the need for further investigation to rule out neoplasia (most often MRI of the course of the facial nerve).

11 Septal perforation

'A 62-year-old man has been referred to your clinic with nasal crusting and a sense of nasal obstruction for a number of years.'

The nasal septum is the division between the left and right nostrils. It is composed of five structures: perpendicular plate of the ethmoid, vomer, cartilage, maxillary crest and palatine crest.

Perforations can be in either the anterior or the posterior part of the septum. They can be asymptomatic or they can cause a number of symptoms – particularly, bleeding, nasal obstruction and nasal whistling.

General structure of the consultation

As always, the structure of the consultation will follow possible causes of the disease. The most common causes are as follows:
+ traumatic causes (e.g. nose picking, external trauma)
+ iatrogenic causes (previous surgery, nasal cautery)
+ inflammatory causes (e.g. sarcoid, Wegener's granulomatosis (WG))
+ infective causes (e.g. syphilis, tuberculosis (TB))
+ neoplastic causes (SCC, basal cell carcinoma, T-cell lymphoma)
+ other causes (chrome workers, illicit drugs such as cocaine).

Specific questions

+ What symptoms are you getting from your nose? (Many perforations are asymptomatic and it is not unusual to diagnose them incidentally when examining the nose for other reasons. Ask specifically about epistaxis, whistling, crusting and sense of nasal obstruction. These are most common with anterior perforations. Posterior perforations are often asymptomatic.)
+ Do you generally have problems with your nose? (Ask specifically about sinusitis, discharge, infections and pain.)
+ Have you had any recent trauma to the nose? (This should include nasal picking and excessively forceful sneezing or blowing of the nose.)
+ Have you had any operations on the nose? (Perforations can arise as a complication of septoplasty and septorhinoplasty.)
+ Have you had recurrent ear infections, sinusitis or chest infections? (This may prompt investigation for WG.)
+ Do you get any problems with your eyes? (Episcleritis and septal pathology may indicate autoimmune disease.)
+ Explore the patient's **I**deas, **C**oncerns and **E**xpectations.

Past medical history and general systems review
◆ Do you have any other medical conditions? (Ask specifically about autoimmune conditions and weight loss, fevers, lethargy and malaise (with neoplasia and granulomatous disease).)

Drug history
◆ Are you on any medications? (Include use of intranasal illicit drugs such as cocaine.)
◆ Any allergies to medications?

Family history
◆ Do any conditions run in the family? (Ask specifically about autoimmune conditions.)

Social history
◆ Do you smoke or drink alcohol?
◆ What do you do for work? (Ascertain whether there has been exposure to noxious substances such as chrome or arsenic.)

Further discussion: explanation and planning
Explain you would perform a full examination of the head and neck, focusing on the nose. Anterior rhinoscopy and rigid endoscopy can be used to delineate limits of perforation and to examine the PNS.

Unless there is an obvious cause, e.g. previous septal surgery, all patients should have baseline blood tests. These include FBC, U+Es (to check renal function, as systemic lupus erythematosus can cause renal failure) and erythrocyte sedimentation rate (ESR)/c-ANCA to assess for autoimmune conditions including WG, angiotensin-converting enzyme (ACE) assay for sarcoidosis and Venereal Disease Research Laboratory test for syphilis.

Other tests include urine dipstick for microscopic haematuria with renal disease, CXR to rule out TB and sarcoidosis, and biopsy, if there is a prominent granular area, to rule out neoplasia.

It is common that investigations do not reveal a cause.

Patients can be a reassured that small septal perforations do not require any additional treatment.

For symptomatic perforations, nasal douching can be used to reduce crusting. If the patient is very troubled by symptoms then consider for surgical repair.

Surgical options: septal button for small anterior perforations. Surgical closure with a number of different flaps has been tried, including with a sliding mucoperichondrial, tunnelled buccal flap. All of these operations have variable rates of success and there is very likely a large inter-surgeon variability in outcomes.

Patients diagnosed with autoimmune or granulomatous disease should be managed in conjunction with immunologist, renal or chest physicians.

12 Hearing loss in a child

> 'A 4-year-old girl comes to your clinic with her mother who is concerned about the child's hearing.'

Neonatal hearing tests within the first few weeks of life are now universal. Congenital hearing loss will most often be picked up at this stage. This often has a genetic basis. Automated otoacoustic emissions (AOAEs) are used as the initial screening test. Those babies who fail the first test (which may or may not be due to an underlying hearing deficit) are retested with AOAEs and automated auditory brainstem responses.

For the purposes of the examination, the most likely scenario will be dealing with hearing loss in older children. The most common cause of hearing impairment in this patient population is OME. This common condition is most often self-limiting, and a period of 6 months' watchful waiting will result in 90% of children spontaneously recovering. However, this is not always the case, and the hearing impairment may compromise speech and language development.

General structure of the consultation

The differential for hearing loss in a child is broad; however, this can be significantly narrowed through careful history taking and examination.

Specific questions

- Has she had recurrent ear infections? (In approximately 50% of OME cases there has been a preceding AOM, particularly in younger children.)
- Has she complained of earache? (Ask also about ear tugging, discharge, fevers, irritability, nausea and poor feeding as signs of AOM.)
- What have you noticed about her hearing? (Ask specifically about interaction with siblings and parents at home, her progress at school and whether she insists on an elevated television volume.)
- Does she snore or have any breathing problems? (Eustachian tube dysfunction may be associated with adenoidal hypertrophy and hence obstructive sleep apnoea and OME.)
- Any recent trauma to the head? (Temporal bone fractures can result in auditory nerve compromise.)
- Any concerns about the development of her speech and language?
- It can be useful to compare development with siblings or peer group. This is a good point to explore the parent's Ideas, Concerns and Expectations.

Past medical history and general systems review

◆ Is she normally well in herself? (Ask about Down's syndrome, cleft palate and other developmental delay that is associated with OME.)
◆ Has she had her routine immunisations?
◆ Was she a full-term baby? (Ask about birth and perinatal history and prematurity, including maternal infections such as TORCH (toxoplasmosis, other, rubella, cytomegalovirus, herpes simplex virus) infections that have been linked to SNHL.)

Drug history

◆ Is she on any medications?
◆ Any allergies to medications?

Family history

◆ Do any conditions run in the family? (Family history of hearing loss/SNHL can have a genetic basis (both recessive and dominant).)

Social history

◆ Is there any smoking in the household? (This has been shown to be associated with OME in children.)

Further discussion: explanation and planning

Explain you would perform full examination of both ears including otoscopy, tympanometry and age-appropriate hearing tests, including air and bone thresholds as appropriate.

Treatment: the most common cause of hearing loss in this population is OME. If clinical signs tally with a corresponding clinical history and type B/C tympanogram and 25 dB hearing loss, then it is reasonable to initially consider a 3-month watchful waiting period. If symptoms are not improving and there is concomitant morbidity (e.g. failure to progress at school), then it may be appropriate to consider surgical management (myringotomy plus grommet insertion, with or without adenoidectomy).

Advice can be given about managing at home and school (e.g. minimising background noise, listening aids in the classroom and working with teaching assistants).

Hearing aids can also be considered.

Genetic screening may be appropriate in patients with SNHL. Plan referral to paediatrician if there is suspicion of a syndromic cause.

Unilateral hearing loss in children is usually managed with lifestyle measures.

Children with bilateral severe to profound SNHL may be considered for cochlear implantation (the indications for implantation are rapidly evolving).

13 Adult with itchy, painful ear

> 'A 50-year-old man has been referred to the ENT casualty clinic with a 2-week history of a painful and itchy left ear. He has tried a number of ear drops from his general practitioner (GP).'

The painful, itchy ear is a very common presentation in ENT outpatient clinics. Routinely, microsuction, symptom control and topical antibiotic therapy are all that is required. However, it is important to remember more sinister causes such as malignant OE.

General structure of the consultation

The most common cause for this presentation in the casualty clinic is OE.

This is defined as an inflammation of the auricle and/or external auditory canal (EAC) up to the medial surface of the TM. It is typically caused by infection, allergy or trauma.

OE can be both acute (under 3 weeks) and chronic (over 3 weeks). The ear canal is often full of tenacious debris, inflamed and narrowed. Presence of inflammatory exudates in the canal can lead to a vicious cycle of exudate, inflammation and pain that is difficult to break. Initially only limited examination may be possible.

Specific questions

- What symptoms are you getting? (Ask specifically about otalgia, discharge, aural fullness and vertigo. If they are getting discharge, ask about the colour, consistency, smell and amount.)
- How long have you had the symptoms?
- What treatment have you received?
- Do you have trouble with the ears frequently and, if so, for how long?
- Do you often get the ears wet? Are you involved in swimming or surfing? (These are typical risk factors for OE.)
- Do you use ear buds to clean your ears or routinely use in-the-ear devices (such as hearing aids or earphones)?
- Have you had any trauma to the ears recently?
- Do you have any allergies? (Patients can develop a type IV hypersensitivity reaction to metals found in earrings such as nickel. Unfortunately, patients can also develop allergies to antibiotics, e.g. topical neomycin.)
- Do you have any other weaknesses or changes in sensation in your body? (It is important to rule out focal neurology, e.g. cranial nerve VII palsy and

severe pain may be indicative of malignant OE (a life-threatening spreading osteomyelitis of the skull base).)

◈ Do you have any pain in the teeth, tonsils, jaw, throat, face or neck? (Pathology outside the ear can be both a cause and a consequence of otalgia due to referred pain.)

Past medical history and general systems review

◈ Do you have any other medical conditions? (Ask specifically about diabetes, which is a risk factor for both benign and malignant OE, and skin conditions such as dermatitis and eczema.)

Drug history

◈ Are you on any medications? (Most patients will have been started on topical antibiotics by the time they are seen in clinic. It is important to find out the type and course length in order to guide appropriate therapy.)
◈ Any allergies to medications?

Family history

◈ Do any conditions run in the family?

Social history

◈ Do you smoke or drink alcohol?
◈ What do you do for work?

Further discussion: explanation and planning

Explain you would perform a full examination of both ears.

Examine for surrounding cellulitis and lymphadenopathy.

Examine mastoids and note any erythema or pinna protrusion. This may signify mastoiditis, although this is extremely rare in adults.

Perform otoscopy – often the canal is filled with debris, which will need to be cleared under microscopic guidance. Middle ear discharge (with underlying perforation) is normally mucoid and can be pulsatile due to middle ear vasculature. It is important to try to completely clear the EAC and to visualise the status of the TM. The quality and consistency of the discharge may signify the infective organism, e.g. offensive, green discharge is typical with Pseudomonas infection. Similarly, it may be possible to visualise fungal hyphae.

Often the EAC is inflamed and narrowed and only minimal suction clearance can be performed. This necessitates the placement of an aural wick for instilment of topical antibiotics. The patient should then be seen in 3–4 days' time for removal of the wick and further attempts at suction clearance.

If otoscopy is normal then it is worth considering the possibility of referred pain (*see* Section 16, Otalgia).

If granulation tissue is seen in the canal, it is prudent to obtain CT imaging, particularly in elderly, immunocompromised patients. MOE is a spreading skull base osteomyelitis that may present with severe otalgia and/or cranial nerve palsies, depending on the extent of the disease. These patients need long-term intravenous antibiotics and, rarely, surgical debridement.

The cornerstones of OE treatment are aural toilet, analgesia and topical antibiotics.

Advise the patient on aural hygiene – particularly regarding keeping the ears dry when showering (vaseline-soaked cotton wool can be useful for this).

Consider topical antibiotics including Sofradex, Otosporin, Otomize or anti-fungals, e.g. clotrimazole solution.

In ongoing infections, a swab should be taken for culture and sensitivity and antibiotics should be chosen on the basis of these.

Acetic acid (Ear Calm) can be useful in controlling symptoms.

There is rarely a need to use systemic antibiotics unless the patient presents with cellulitis or MOE or is immunocompromised.

14 Adult with non-acute hearing loss

'A 54-year-old man is brought to the ENT clinic by his wife who is fed up having to shout to be heard at home.'

Hearing loss is extremely common in the general adult population. It can range from extremely mild to profound loss with subsequent impact on social functioning. Approximately 10% of the adult population has some degree of hearing loss; however, this rises to 35% in the age group over 65 years. Hearing loss can result from impairment to any part of the auditory pathway, from the auricle to the CNS. Gradual hearing loss in the adult tends to be sensorineural in origin resulting from lesions of the inner ear or vestibulocochlear nerve (cranial nerve VIII).

General structure of the consultation

This is a common presentation in ENT clinic. The key to making a diagnosis is in the history. The majority of these patients will have idiopathic SNHL. However, it is worth remembering other identifiable causes, e.g. infections, neoplasia, trauma, neurological reasons, metabolic reasons, toxicity and autoimmune reasons.

Specific questions

- What have you noticed about your hearing?
- How severe is the loss and how is it affecting your day-to-day activities?
- Did it come on gradually or suddenly? (Try to ascertain the exact circumstances when the hearing loss was noticed.)
- How was your hearing before?
- Is it one ear or both ears?
- Have you had problems with your ears in the past? (Ask specifically about tinnitus, fullness, dizziness, pain, discharge and wax problems.)
- Any recent coughs or colds? (These may predispose to OME.)
- Have you had any recent chest infections, sinusitis or kidney problems? (This screens for autoimmune conditions and granulomatous disease that can present with hearing loss and systemic symptoms.)
- Do you have any problems with your nose? (Ask about discharge, epistaxis and obstruction. This screens for PNS lesions that are associated with OME.)
- Any weaknesses or changes in sensation? (Cranial nerve lesions are a feature of advanced neoplasia.)

◆ Any recent trauma to your head? (Temporal bone fractures can disrupt the auditory pathways.)

Past medical history and general systems review

◆ Do you have any other medical conditions? (Ask specifically about autoimmune conditions and weight loss, fevers, lethargy, malaise (with neoplasia and granulomatous disease), hypertension, hyperlipidaemia and exposure to infectious agents, e.g. syphilis or HIV.

Drug history

◆ Are you on any medications? (A number of drugs are associated with hearing loss, particularly aminoglycoside antibiotics, platinum chemotherapeutic agents and loop diuretics.)
◆ Any allergies to medications?

Family history

◆ Do any conditions run in the family? (Hearing loss may be heritable (many deafness-related genes have been cloned; disease such as otosclerosis cluster in families).)

Social history

◆ Do you smoke or drink alcohol?
◆ What do you do for work? (Ask about noise exposure.)

Further discussion: explanation and planning

Explain you would perform a full examination of both ears including otoscopy, PTA and tympanogram.

If findings are suggestive of OME, examine the PNS to rule out any neoplasia, e.g. nasopharyngeal carcinoma.

If there are other 'red flag' symptoms such as unilateral hearing loss or tinnitus, vertigo or vestibular symptoms, then intracranial imaging may be appropriate.

Plan investigation for autoimmune/granulomatous disease, depending on history.

Most hearing loss in adults will be SNHL associated with presbycusis – consider referral to audiology care. Hearing loss in this population is often managed with hearing aids.

15 Adult with sudden hearing loss

'A 29-year-old man is referred by his GP with a history of unilateral hearing loss for 72 hours.'

General structure of the consultation

A sudden SNHL is defined as a loss of 30 dB or more, over at least three contiguous audiometric frequencies that develops over 3 days or less in an ear with previously normal hearing or a decrease in hearing in an ear with a pre-existing loss. The most usual aetiology is a sensorineural loss, although conductive losses can presently similarly. The majority of cases are idiopathic; however, there are some important treatable causes that must be ruled out.

Specific questions

- How did you notice the hearing loss?
- How severe is it?
- Did the hearing loss come on gradually or suddenly? (Many patients notice hearing loss when they wake up in the morning or when trying to use the telephone with that ear.)
- How was your hearing before? (Hearing loss can occur in previously normal ears, ears with a pre-existing hearing impairment or as part of a disorder with fluctuating hearing levels, such as Ménière's syndrome.)
- Is the hearing loss in one ear or in both ears? (Three per cent of acoustic neuromas present with sudden hearing loss.)
- Do you have any other symptoms? (Ask specifically about vertigo, tinnitus, wax problems and discharge.)
- Screen for the patient's **I**deas, **C**oncerns and **E**xpectations.

Past medical history and general systems review

- Do you have any other medical conditions? (Systemic diseases including multiple sclerosis, antiphospholipid syndrome and autoimmune diseases could theoretically present initially with sudden hearing loss. Ask about neurological conditions – such as drop attacks, transient loss of consciousness, neck pain, weaknesses, paraesthesias, vertigo and double vision – as these can be the presentation of vertebrobasilar insufficiency.)
- Have you been diagnosed with a cancer or tumour in the past? (Sudden hearing loss can be caused post irridation and as an effect of chemotherapy agents such as cisplatin.)

◆ Have you been exposed to any loud sounds or any recent head trauma? (A perilymph fistula should be considered if there is a history of pressure changes and sudden hearing loss associated with a positive fistula test (nystagmus when applying manual pressure to the ipsilateral tragus).)

Drug history

◆ Are you on any medications? (It is important to take a full drug history, as there are some commonly used ototoxic medications – particularly, platinum-based chemotherapy, aminoglycoside antibiotics, salicylates and loop diuretics.)
◆ Any allergies to medications?

Family history

◆ Do any conditions run in the family?

Social history

◆ Have you been travelling recently? (Ask about foreign travel and travel to areas with endemic Lyme disease.)
◆ Ascertain a sexual history. HIV and syphilis are associated with sudden hearing loss.

Further discussion: explanation and planning

Explain you would perform a full ear examination including otoscopy to exclude any conductive losses such as OME or wax.

Plan a full examination of cranial nerves – hearing loss with other focal neurology may suggest a vascular/neoplastic origin, e.g. paraesthesia in distribution of cranial nerve V with acoustic neuromas or diplopia with cranial nerve VI involvement.

Perform a fistula test if the history is suggestive of a perilymphatic fistula.

Perform PTA/tympanometry to get an objective measure of the hearing loss.

Blood tests should be ordered in correspondence with the clinical history and examination findings. For example, HbA1c in suspected diabetes or FBC, ESR or autoimmune antibody screen if autoimmune pathology is suspected.

In unilateral hearing loss, gadolinium contrast MRI is the most useful examination of the internal acoustic meatus for acoustic neuroma.

Treatment is decided on the basis of clinical findings. There is no obvious cause in the majority of cases. This should be explained to the patient.

Numerous treatment regimens including steroids, plasma expanders, aciclovir and carbogen have been tried; however, the evidence remains inconclusive.

A number of studies have pointed to the benefit of a short, high-dose regimen of oral corticosteroids for sudden unilateral hearing loss (a commonly used protocol is 1 mg/kg prednisolone for 7 days). Patients should be informed of the risk involved with taking steroids, such as disturbed sleep and gastric ulceration.

Arrange to follow up with the patient in 4–6 weeks to repeat hearing tests and to monitor progress.

In cases where there is no improvement, hearing aids may be considered, particularly in bilateral cases (often no treatment is required in unilateral cases).

Patients must be informed that they need to seek urgent medical attention if they experience hearing loss in the contralateral ear, as immediate treatment is very likely to be warranted.

16 Otalgia

'A 30-year-old man is referred to the ENT clinic with a 3-month history of left-sided ear pain.'

General structure of the consultation

Otalgia is a complicated presenting complaint because of the multiplicity of causative factors. Pain can be of otological (outer, middle or inner ear) or non-otological origin. Careful history taking and examination is required to discern these.

Specific questions

- When did the pain start?
- Is it getting better or worse?
- What makes it better or worse?
- Do you notice any other symptoms with the pain?
- Do you have any problems with your teeth?
- Do you have any problems with your nose? (Ask specifically about rhinorrhea, obstruction, catarrh and post-nasal drip, as rhinosinusitis associated with Eustachian tube dysfunction can present as otalgia.)
- Any recent coughs and colds? (Odynophagia with referred otalgia is commonly associated with infections of the upper aerodigestive tract such as tonsillitis and pharyngitis, but also with neoplastic disease.)
- Do you get heartburn or reflux? (Reflux can be associated with otalgia.)
- Do you have any pain or limitation in movement of the neck? (This can imply referred otalgia is due to the irritation of the upper cervical nerve roots.)

Past medical history and general systems review

- Do you have any other conditions? (Ask specifically about hypertension, diabetes.)
- Have you been diagnosed with a cancer or tumour in the past? (Metastatic disease from other head and neck primary sites is possible.)

Drug history

- Are you on any medications?
- Any allergies to medications?

Family history

◆ Do any conditions run in the family?

Further discussion: explanation and planning

Explain you would perform a full examination of the ear.

Full examination of the cranial nerves is very important, as other neurological signs may be indicative of a space-occupying lesion. For example, lesions of the petrous apex V/VI deficit, lower cranial nerve lesions in metastatic tumours of the pharynx/larynx, VII nerve palsy in parotid gland malignancy.

Examine the dentition and temporomandibular joints.

Examine the cervical spine for joint tenderness, neck movements and muscle spasms.

Other investigations include orthopantogram (dental X-ray), barium swallow, panendoscopy and biopsy.

In high-risk cases, CT of the head and neck may be indicated to rule out malignancy, particularly in areas difficult to detect clinically such as the tongue base and tonsil.

17 Nasal crusting

'A 42-year-old woman attends the ENT clinic with a history of "always having loads of stuff up my nose".'

General structure of the consultation

This is a common presentation in ENT clinics and in the general population. In the majority of cases it requires no specific treatment. However, there are systemic conditions that can present with nasal crusting, so a thorough history is required. A chronic presentation without systemic symptoms is very likely to have a local cause such as atrophic rhinitis, trauma or rhinosinusitis.

Specific questions

- What exact problems are you having with your nose? (It is important to ask open questions initially, particularly when the presenting complaint is quite vague.)
- How long have you been having problems?
- Do you have any other problems with the nose? (It is important to ask about nasal obstruction, which can be associated with polyps.)
- Do you have nasal whistling or changes in the 'gristle' of the nose? (This may indicate a septal perforation with overlying crust.)
- Do you have nosebleeds, facial weakness, sensory changes, changes in vision, facial pain or headaches? (These may be suggestive of underlying sinonasal malignancy.)
- Do you have any disturbance in your sense of smell? (Olfactory dysfunction – cacosmia may be indicative of atrophic rhinitis.)
- Ask about nasal picking. (This is the leading cause of septal perforation.)
- Have you had any other nasal trauma? (This includes nasogastric tube insertions and irradiation.)
- Do you have any problems with your ears? (An associated OME may be a sign of a nasopharyngeal malignancy but it may also indicate vasculitides such as Churg–Strauss syndrome (CS).)
- Do you have any hearing loss? (WG can cause a SNHL or mixed hearing loss.)

Past medical history and general systems review

- Do you have any other medical conditions? (A full systems review is required in all cases as vasculitis and granulomatosis disease that can present with nasal crusting have manifestations in all areas of the body. Ask specifically about haematuria, haemoptysis, shortness of breath, paraesthesia, weaknesses and changes in vision.)

◈ Have you had any previous operations on the nose? (Particularly mention septoplasty and submucous resection.)

Drug history

◈ Are you on any medications? (Include intranasal cocaine, as this can cause widespread nasal damage because of its vasoconstrictive properties, as can home oxygen use through drying of the nasal mucosa and repeated trauma from nasal prongs.)

◈ Any allergies to medications?

Family history

◈ Do any conditions run in the family?

Social history

◈ Ask about travel history and ethnic heritage. (TB, acquired immune deficiency syndrome, syphilis, rhinoscleroma and leprosy are possible causes and the relevant investigations should be performed in at-risk individuals.)

◈ What do you do for work? (Ask about exposure to chrome salts. Workers in leather and nickel industries are particularly at risk. Woodworkers are at risk from sinonasal malignancy (most frequently, adenocarcinoma).)

Further discussion: explanation and planning

A full examination of the nose should be undertaken using anterior rhinoscopy and rigid endoscopy. The areas of nasal crusting should be noted. The septum should be examined for perforations. Any suspicious areas should be biopsied (particularly irregular or granulating mucosa).

Plan to examine for fetor and polyps.

Granulomatous disease such as WG causes irregular 'cobblestone' oedematous mucosa.

CS predisposes to polyps and allergic rhinitis.

Plan a full examination of the ears including PTA/tympanometry if indicated.

Treatment depends on the cause – in post-traumatic cases it is very likely that no treatment is appropriate.

If systemic features are detected in the history, a range of investigations may be appropriate. These include cANCA/pANCA (WG/CS), ACE levels (sarcoidosis), urinalysis/CXR (WG), and FBC/U+Es (anaemia is associated with sarcoidosis and eosinophilia is associated with CS).

Plan a nasal septal biopsy if neoplasia is suspected.

Plan referral to other specialities where systemic disease is suspected, e.g. WG patients are usually managed under the joint care of respiratory, renal and ENT physicians.

Further treatment includes nasal irrigation and humidification.

Surgical treatment involves repair of septal perforation. Radical procedures (e.g. Young's operation) are less popular.

18 Dizziness

'A 28-year-old woman attends the ENT clinic complaining of feeling dizzy.'

General structure of the consultation

The complexity of the vestibular system coupled with the often non-specific symptoms of the patients make evaluating the dizzy patient a difficult consultation. However, with a careful history it is possible to differentiate the important causes and often to provide appropriate therapy. Ultimately, you must distinguish between true vertigo and imbalance and peripheral from central causes of vertigo.

Specific questions

- Please explain to me what is happening when you are dizzy. (Differentiate between true vertigo ('the room spins'), disequilibrium (impaired gait), presyncope (the feeling of faintness) and general non-specific 'light-headedness'. In dizzy patients without true vertigo, an underlying medical cause such as cardiac arrhythmia needs to be ruled out. For the purposes of the ENT clinic, we will focus on the patients with true vertigo.)
- Tell me about the first time you became dizzy. (Allow the patient to speak without interrupting her. This will elucidate the time course of the onset of the dizziness and will suggest a cause of acute vestibular failure that may not be clear from the rest of the history.)
- Are you always dizzy or does it come in episodes?
- Tell me more about an episode.
- How often do the episodes come and how long do they last? (Short, self-terminating episodes that are positionally determined (e.g. turning over in bed) suggest benign paroxysmal positional vertigo (BPPV). Longer episodes are suggestive of vestibular failure (e.g. in a Ménière's syndrome crisis). Continued vertigo is suggestive of central causes, e.g. multiple sclerosis.)
- Is there anything you can do to make it better? (Ask if visual fixation improves the vertigo. A peripheral cause for vertigo is improved, while a central vertigo is unaffected.)
- Is there anything you have noticed that brings on the vertigo? (Ask about characteristic head positions for BPPV and the occurrence of vertigo with loud sounds (Tullio's phenomenon) that may indicate an underlying superior canal dehiscence.)
- Have you noticed associated symptoms? (Particularly, enquire about hearing

loss, tinnitus, aural discharge and pyrexia. A presentation of episodic low-tone hearing loss, aural fullness, tinnitus and vertigo is pathognomic of Ménière's syndrome. Vertigo with 'aura' such as visual or olfactory disturbance and headache is classic of migranous vertigo. Vertigo with asymmetric hearing loss and/or tinnitus could be a result of a vestibular schwannoma (a rare presenting symptom).

◈ Were you unwell before the first episode of dizziness? (Viral infections predispose to vestibular failure.)

Past medical history and general systems review

◈ Do you have any other medical conditions? (Ask about general health including cardiovascular disease, diabetes, eye problems and mobility or joint problems – these conditions often manifest as imbalance.)

◈ Have you had any recent trauma to the head? (Temporal bone fractures can involve the vestibular system.)

◈ Have you had any previous surgery to the ears?

◈ Explore the patient's Ideas, Concerns and Expectations. Specifically, explore the patient's fear around the possibility of brain tumours. This is very likely to be what the patient is worried about.

Drug history

◈ Are you on any medications? (Ask about use of antibiotics. For example, gentamicin is known to be toxic to both the vestibular and the cochlear systems. Antihypertensives cause positional hypotension, an important cause of disequilibrium particularly in the elderly. It is important that multiple medications and multiple co-morbidities in the elderly lead to multifactorial dizziness.)

◈ Any allergies to medications?

Family history

◈ Do any conditions run in the family? (Ask about Ménière's syndrome.)

Social history

◈ Do you smoke or drink alcohol? (Ask about relation of these activities to the symptoms.)

◈ What do you do for work? (Ask about the effect of the symptoms on their ability to do their job safely. This is important if they drive for a living.)

◈ Ask about stress. (Vertigo can be a psychogenic condition that improves with stress management techniques.)

◈ Are you currently driving? (They may need to contact the Driver and Vehicle Licensing Agency for advice as to whether it is appropriate for them to continue to do so.)

Further discussion: explanation and planning

Explain that you will need to examine their ears, eyes and sense of balance with some simple tests.

Lying and standing blood pressures should be taken. A significant postural drop may indicate the true cause of the patient's symptoms.

Perform a standard examination of the ear. This is to rule out any middle ear disease, e.g. OME or cholesteatoma. Perform a fistula test.

Assess for the presence of nystagmus. A horizontal nystagmus is typical of a peripheral vertigo. Vertical nystagmus indicates a central cause. The direction of the nystagmus is classically described in terms of the direction of the fast phase.

Perform a head thrust test. In acute vestibular failure, the vestibulo-ocular response fails and fixation is lost.

Perform a full examination of all other cranial nerves. Gross signs are often obvious but subtler signs, such as a V nerve palsy manifesting as a loss of corneal reflex with a vestibular schwannoma, is easier to miss.

Perform balance tests – Unterberger's and Romberg's tests can reveal gross derangements in equilibrium, but they are not specific in differentiating central from peripheral lesions.

Perform a Dix–Hallpike procedure for BPPV (there are numerous videos available online for more information on this procedure).

Inform the patient that you will formally assess their hearing with a pure-tone audiogram.

Imaging is indicated in patients with unilateral symptoms, e.g. vertigo with unilateral tinnitus or SNHL. In most units the imaging of choice is MRI, primarily to exclude vestibular schwannomas but also to examine the CNS for other conditions, such as brainstem plaques in multiple sclerosis.

Other tests such as the caloric test are not often performed in routine clinical practice.

Treatment will depend on the underlying condition. Patients with acute vestibular failure should be reassured and informed that their condition will improve naturally. They should be directed to a trustworthy balance information source for vestibular rehabilitation exercises if the balance disorder continues. Vestibular sedatives may be of use in the acute phase.

In patients with a positive Dix–Hallpike result, an Epley procedure can be performed in clinic. This procedure has a high success rate in BPPV and it can be repeated. Patients can also be taught how to perform the procedure at home (there are a number of training aids available, e.g. DizzyFIX).

The management of Ménière's syndrome remains controversial. Many patients find the adoption of a low-sodium diet useful. Caffeine and tobacco have also been suggested as exacerbating factors. There is equivocal evidence for treatment with diuretics. Crises can be treated with vestibular sedatives and antiemetics. In severe cases, the patient may opt for ablative therapy (intratympanic gentamicin, endolymphatic sac surgery, labyrinthectomy, vestibular nerve section).

19 Neck lump

'A 58-year-old man attends the ENT clinic after noticing a lump in his neck.'

General structure of the consultation

Neck lumps are common both in examinations and in clinical practice. In children they are normally a benign reactive lymphadenopathy; in adults the majority are malignant. There are a number of potential causes and the likelihood of each depends on the patient demographic and the history.

Common causes include:

- Congenital (seen in children and adults)
  - branchial cyst
  - thyroglossal cyst
  - laryngocele
  - teratoma
  - dermoid cyst
  - cystic hygroma
- Infective (seen in adults and children)
  - viral lymphadenopathy
  - bacterial lymphadenopathy
  - granulomatous disease, e.g. sarcoid, TB
- Neoplastic (particularly in adults)
  - metastatic SCC
  - thyroid masses
  - lymphoma
- Vascular (particularly in adults)
  - carotid aneurysm
  - carotid body tumour.

Specific questions

- When did you first notice the lump? (A short history, single, firm, lateral lump: often malignant or reactive. A short history, multiple, rubbery lumps: lymphoma, glandular fever, TB. A longer history, single and lateral lump: branchial cyst. A longer history, single, midline lump: thyroid mass, thyroglossal cyst.)
- Is it getting larger? (Malignant nodes tend to enlarge rapidly. Infective nodes often accompany a URTI.)

- Do you have any nasal blockage? (This can be associated with lesions in the PNS, e.g. nasopharyngeal carcinoma.)
- Any pain in the ears? (Head and neck primaries often present with otalgia.)
- Any pain in the throat? (Can be associated with head and neck primaries, and also with infective conditions such as glandular fever and tonsillitis.)
- Have you noticed any change in your voice? (Voice change and hoarseness are a 'red flag' for neoplasia.)
- Have you had any trouble swallowing? (Pharyngeal lesions may mechanically obstruct swallowing.)
- Do you smoke cigarettes?
- Do you drink alcohol? (Alcohol and smoking are risk factors for head and neck neoplasia.)
- Have you lost any weight? (Weight loss is associated with neoplasia (SCC, lymphoma) and infective conditions such as TB.)
- How is your appetite?
- Have you had any night sweats?
- Have you had any fevers? (Fevers and night sweats are associated with lymphoma and infective conditions such as TB.)
- Have you had any holidays abroad lately? (A risk factor for TB.)
- Have you had a recent chest infection or URTI? (A very common cause of reactive lymphadenopathy.)
- Does the lump change with eating? (Salivary masses often change with eating.)

Past medical history and general systems review
- Do you have any other medical conditions? (Ask about general health including cardiovascular disease and diabetes.)
- Explore the patient's **I**deas, **C**oncerns and **E**xpectations.

Drug history
- Are you on any medications?
- Any allergies to medications?

Family history
- Do any conditions run in the family?

Social history
- What do you do for work? (Check for exposure to chemicals and animals, e.g. abattoir work may propose to rare infections such as brucellosis.)

Further discussion: explanation and planning

Explain that you will perform a full ENT examination. This will include examination of the PNS, base of tongue, tonsils, pharynx, larynx and thyroid.

Examine the lump for size, site, character, pulsatility, mobility and transillumination.

Perform FNA (for microbiology and cytology). This can be under USS guidance.

Plan blood tests including FBC, white cell count, ESR and c-reactive protein.

Special tests are Infectious Mononucleosis screen, HIV, CXR, barium swallow (with any dysphagia), CT of the head and neck/chest (for staging if the lump is very likely to be neoplastic).

Panendoscopy is indicated if there is a high index of suspicion for malignant disease and the original examination was unable to locate a primary. Blind biopsies of the PNS, tongue base, tonsils and piriform fossae can aid in diagnosis.

CHAPTER 2

Examination Stations

The DO-HNS examination demands a fluent and confident approach to the basic ENT, head and neck examination. It is of the upmost importance to have a logical system for examining the ear, nose and neck, as these are most commonly tested in the examination.

Marks in the examination are primarily given for the form and comprehensiveness of the examination rather than for the signs elicited. You might find it helpful to talk through what you are doing and what you have found as you go. Some examiners will require you to do this, although most stay relatively passive and allow you to continue with the examination at your own pace.

The general examination schema learnt in medical school inspection, palpation and auscultation holds true here too. This needs to be modified for the head and neck examination, as palpation and auscultation play smaller roles than in other body systems.

General rules for examinations:

- Always introduce yourself and gain consent and cooperation of the patient. A good opening may be: 'Hello, I am Dr Jones. Would it be OK if I examined your ears and hearing?'
- Always enquire whether the patient is currently in any pain. It is not professional to cause patients pain in examinations or in clinical practice.

Tips for success in the examination stations:

- Design a scheme for examining the ear, the nose and the neck. Make sure that it has a logical order, covers all the important areas and that you can remember it.
- Practise your schemes at every opportunity. You do not always need patients with clinical signs for this.

◆ Recognise that in the examination you will be feeling nervous and stressed. The more practice you do, the less nervy you will be when it comes to the examination. If you do forget something it is very rarely 'fatal', as you will have picked up plenty of marks elsewhere.

◆ Before and after you touch any patient, use the alcohol gel provided. There are lots of easy marks going for this.

◆ Make sure you are bare below the elbows. Men should not wear ties (in examinations).

◆ Stay calm – things are just easier that way.

1 Examination of the ear

This is the most important examination scheme to master for the DO-HNS examination. In short, you can be guaranteed that you will be tested on examining the ear. Get practising – repetition is most definitely the key to success. Remember examining normal ears is beneficial, as it makes detecting pathology much easier. Often there is no pathology to see in the examination; however, the actors often fabricate a hearing loss to be picked up using the objective tests described in this section.

Introduce yourself to the patient. Explain that you are going to be examining their ears and hearing: 'Hello, I am Dr Jones. I understand you have been having some trouble with your ears. Would it be OK if I could examine your ears and hearing?'

Clean your hands with the alcohol gel. Feel free to stress the importance of infection control.

Tell the patient that you will be explaining to them what you are doing as you go along, but let them know to ask if they have any questions. Explaining the findings to the patient shows good rapport. In older style examinations, candidates had to present their findings at the end of the examination. This is not usual practice in the DO-HNS examination, where the focus is primarily on procedure and completeness rather than on the findings.

Ask which is their 'better' ear.

Ask if they are currently in any pain. This is extremely important. If the patient indicates they have pain from one ear then it should be examined with care.

Test your otoscope to check that it is working and then commence inspection of the better ear (using the light from the otoscope).

Areas to look at:

- pinna (scars, quality of cartilage, active infections, compare symmetry with the other side)
- mastoid (move the pinna forwards, asking again about pain)
- preauricular area (look for pits, sinuses, fistulae)
- conchal bowl.

Now proceed with examining the other ear and make a comparison between them.

Now proceed to examine the external auditory canal (EAC) and tympanic membrane (TM) with the otoscope (held in the same hand as the ear you are examining, between the thumb and forefinger). For this you will need to pull the pinna posterosuperiorly to straighten the canal with the other hand. Choose the largest speculum that fits into the canal to give the best view of the TM.

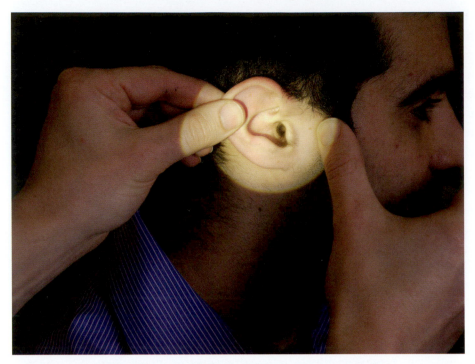

FIGURE 2.1 Examining the ear, pulling the pinna posterosuperiorly

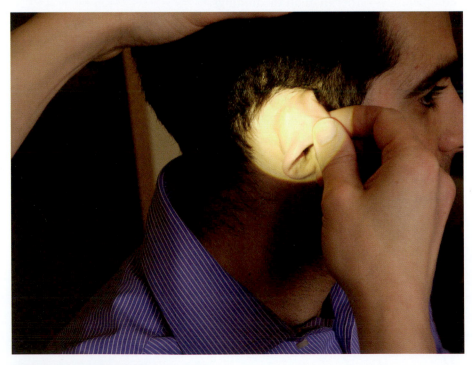

FIGURE 2.2 Examining the mastoid

You should use the little finger of the hand holding the otoscope to brace against the cheek of the patient; this should stop any damage to the ear if the patient makes any sudden movement.

Be gentle with the otoscope. Make sure when you are moving it around in the EAC that your movements are slow and considered, otherwise you will cause the patient pain. In the examination the 'patient' will have had their ears examined a number of times before, hence their tolerance to any sudden movements is quite low.

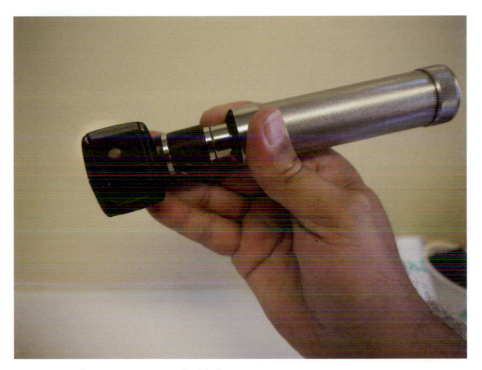

FIGURE 2.3 The correct way to hold the otoscope

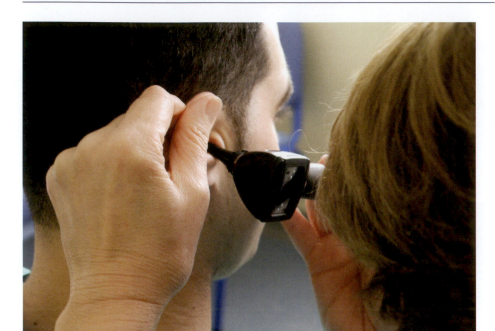

FIGURE 2.4 Examining the ear using the otoscope

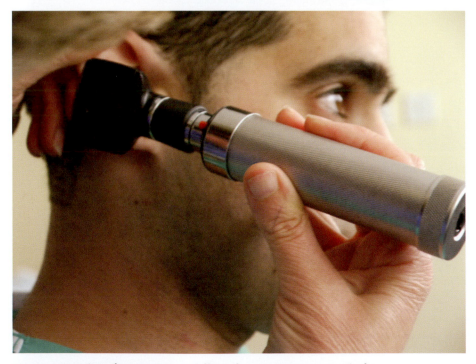

FIGURE 2.5 Using the otoscope, pulling the ear posterosuperiorly

Areas to comment on:

◈ EAC (look for discharge, bony swellings)
◈ pars tensa (any perforations, retraction pockets, ossicles – particularly the lateral process of malleus and long process of incus, presence of grommets)
◈ pars flaccida (attic retraction pockets, cholesteatoma)

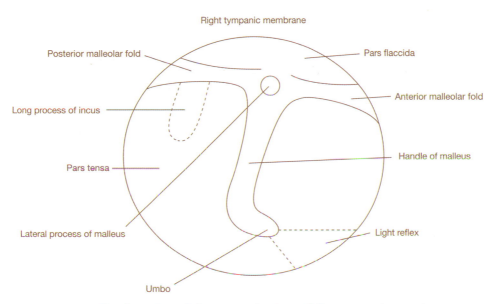

FIGURE 2.6 A stylised version of the otoscopic view of the tympanic membrane

At this point, indicate to the examiner that you would usually perform pneumatic otoscopy to assess the mobility of the TM.

Next, perform the fistula test – apply tragal pressure and watch the eyes for nystagmus with a fast phase away from the diseased side. This test is positive with a lateral semicircular fistula. This step can be omitted if the rubric specifies not to examine the balance system.

Next, explain to the patient that you are going to perform some tests of their hearing. (NB. These tests are often not performed if there is easy access to an audiology department that can perform an audiogram; however, these tests remain useful when audiology is not available.)

First, perform a free field test of the patient's hearing.

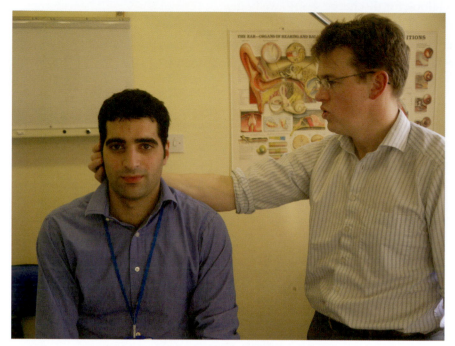

FIGURE 2.7 Performance of free field hearing test at 60 cm

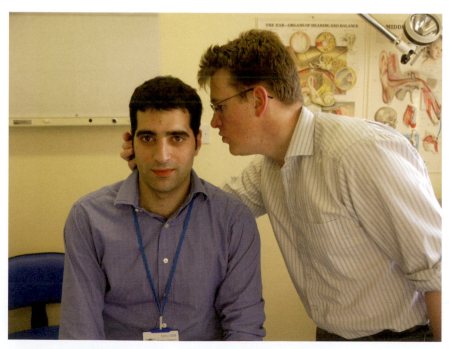

FIGURE 2.8 Performance of free field hearing test at 15 cm

The non-test ear is masked with tragal pressure and the patient's eyes are shielded to prevent any visual stimulus. Do not place your arm across the face of the patient when masking the contralateral ear. It is far nicer for the patient to occlude the ear from behind their head.

You will then whisper three two-syllable words or bi-digit numbers from 60 cm from the test ear. If the patient gets two out of these three correct then the hearing level is 12 dB or better.

If there is no accurate response, use a conversational voice (48 dB or worse) or a loud voice (76 dB or worse).

You can then move closer and repeat the test at 15 cm. Here the thresholds are 34 dB for a whisper and 56 dB for a conversational voice.

Next, perform Rinne's and Weber's tests. There will be a number of tuning forks laid out on the examination table. Always choose the 512 Hz fork (and make sure the examiner has seen you do this!). This gives the best balance between time of decay and tactile vibration (ideally, you want a fork that has a long period of decay and cannot be detected by vibration sensation).

Explain to the patient that you are going to be testing their hearing using the tuning forks.

Perform Weber's test first, by placing a 512 Hz tuning fork in the midline forehead or the vertex. The tuning fork should be set in motion by striking it on your knee (not on the patient's knee or a table). Ask the patient whether they hear it loudest in the right, the left or the middle and note the result.

Next, perform Rinne's test. Place a vibrating 512 Hz tuning fork firmly on the test ear mastoid process (apply pressure to the opposite side of the head to make sure the contact is firm, ideally from behind so you are not shielding the patient's eyes with your hands, as many patients find this claustrophobic). It is very important that the fork goes on to the mastoid process. It is surprising the number of people who do not perform this correctly. If you are unsure, it is wise to get one of your consultants to show you how best to do this. The examiners will certainly check the fork is correctly placed.

This tests the bone conduction. Next, place the tuning fork in front of the test ear with the tuning fork's tines perpendicular to the head, hence testing air conduction. Ask the patient which they heard loudest and take note of the result.

A positive Rinne's test result is NORMAL, where the air conduction is heard better than the bone conduction. This is unusual for a medical sign, where the positive sign is usually pathological. This can lead to some confusion. Normal hearing will have a positive Rinne's test result in both ears and Weber's test will be central.

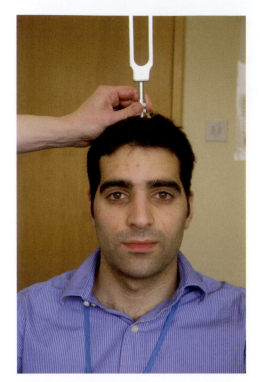

FIGURE 2.9 Weber's test

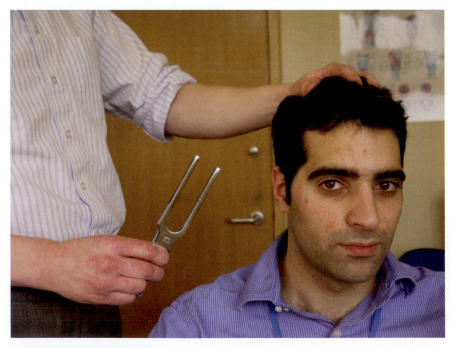

FIGURE 2.10 Rinne's test

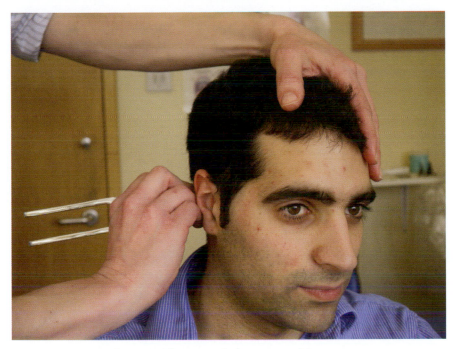

FIGURE 2.11 Rinne's test with tuning fork on mastoid process

You should present the findings to the examiner as you detected them and then interpret the findings to give a diagnosis if there is any hearing loss.

TABLE 2.1 Findings from Rinne's and Weber's tests (AC = air conduction, BC = bone conduction)

	Weber lateralises left	Weber lateralises right
Rinne positive both ears AC > BC	Sensorineural loss in right	Sensorineural loss in left
Rinne negative left BC > AC	Conductive loss in left	Sensorineural loss in left
Rinne negative right BC > AC	Sensorineural loss in right	Conductive loss in right

This completes the examination of the ear for the purpose of the DO-HNS examination.

To complete your examination, tell the examiner you would like to examine all the cranial nerves, paying particular attention to the facial nerve. Any facial nerve weakness should be graded on the House–Brackmann scale (I–VI). You would also like to examine the post-nasal space with a rigid endoscope, paying particular attention to the openings of the Eustachian tubes, where nasopharyngeal carcinomas can arise.

You would also send the patient for formal audiological examination including PTA and tympanometry.

Thank the patient for their cooperation and use the alcohol gel as you leave.

EXAMINATION PEARL

A useful phrase to remember the scheme:

Inspection-Something (fistula test)-**Hearing tests-Something** (facial nerve and PNS)

Another useful memory jog is the four Fs:

Fields, Forks, Fistula, Facial nerve

Example ear examination mark scheme (each point scored to a maximum of 4 points)

- Introduction
- Consent, cooperation, suitable exposure
- Explanation of procedure
- Reassurance
- Correct use of otoscope (including checking it works)
- Inspection of both ears including EACs/TMs
- Tuning fork tests
- Free field hearing tests
- Fistula test
- Suggestion of extra test (cranial nerves, audio, balance system)

2 Examination of the nose

Introduce yourself and explain to the patient that you are going to be examining their nose: 'Hello, I am Dr Jones. Would it be OK if I could examine your nose and sinuses?'

Ask if they currently have any pain in their nose or face. Proceed with care if they indicate that they currently have tender areas.

Sit facing the patient with your knees together and to one side of the patient's knees. It is not pleasant for the patient to be 'straddled'.

Start by gelling your hands and then inspect the nose from the front while seated. Then you can stand and examine the nose from above, below and each side.

Areas to comment on:

◆ nasal dorsum (saddling, erythema, scars, dorsal hump)

◆ tip (any depression, ptosis, over-projection)

◆ columella (gently elevate the tip to check for columella dislocation).

Inspect the face, commenting particularly on the presence of any rash (infection, autoimmune disease).

Next, take the Thudicum's speculum and carefully examine each side of the nose in turn. Make sure you are familiar with how to hold the speculum. The correct method is slightly counter-intuitive but allows the best visualisation

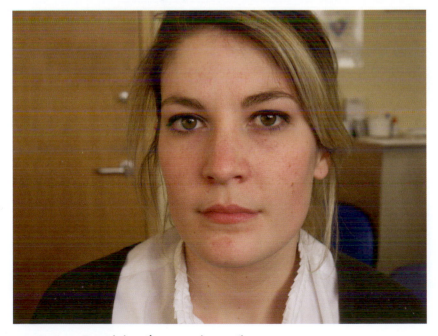

FIGURE 2.12 Examining the nose, inspection

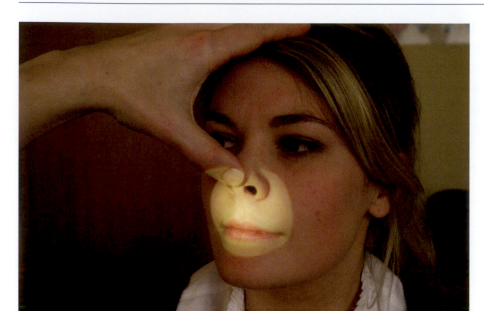

FIGURE 2.13 Examining the nasal vestibules with columella retraction

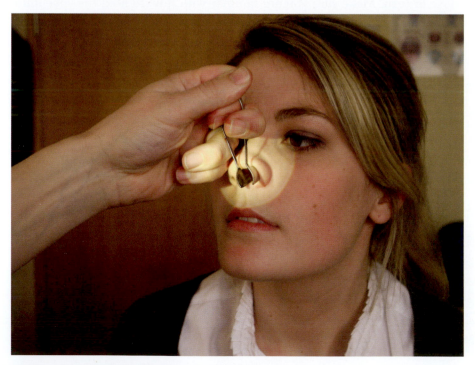

FIGURE 2.14 Use of the Thudicum's speculum

of the nasal mucosa. Insert your index finger into the bend of the speculum and support it above with the thumb. The middle and ring fingers are used to manipulate the tines of the speculum. You are effectively looking through the gap between these two fingers.

Areas to comment on:

◆ septum (perforations, deviations, mucosal damage, areas of cautery)
◆ lateral wall (size of turbinates, polyps).

Next, perform an examination of the nasal airflow by asking the patient to exhale while holding a Lack's metallic tongue depressor under the nose. Assess the pattern of fogging on the depressor.

Ask the patient to sniff in and watch for evidence of vestibular collapse.

If there is any nasal obstruction, perform Cottle's test by applying lateral pressure to the cheek at the side of the nose to see whether this improves the nasal airway (a positive Cottle's test indicates nasal valve stenosis).

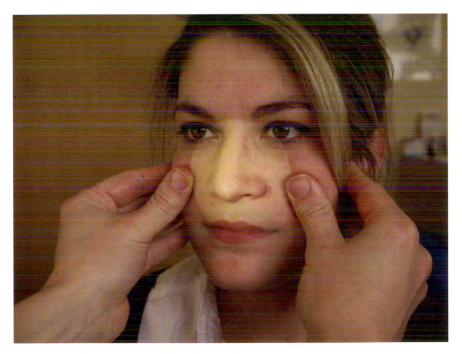

FIGURE 2.15 Performance of Cottle's test

Examine the oropharynx, soft palate and upper teeth (*see* Section 4, Examination of the oral cavity).

Suggest to the examiner that you would like to examine the nose and PNS

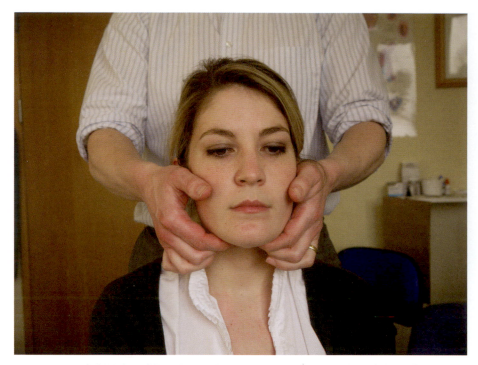

FIGURE 2.20 Palpation of level 1 nodes

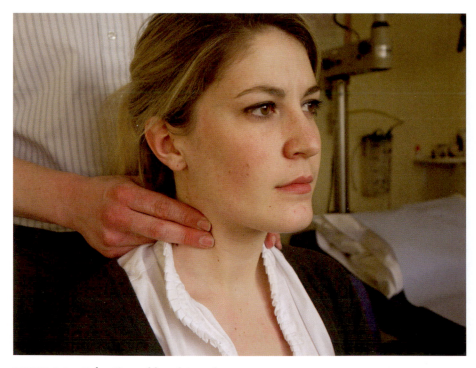

FIGURE 2.21 Palpation of level 2 nodes

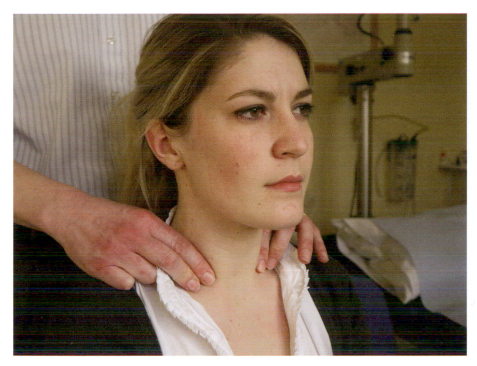

FIGURE 2.22 Palpation of level 3 and 4 nodes

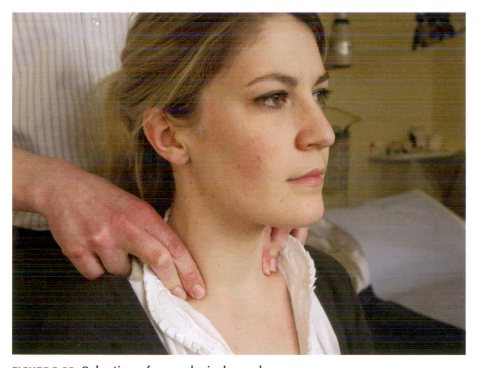

FIGURE 2.23 Palpation of supraclavicular nodes

Move on to examining the eyes – check for lid lag and for loss of hair from the outer third of the eyebrows.

Check for chemosis and exophthalmos.

Percuss the upper sternum for retrosternal extension.

You can also suggest you would examine the legs for pretibial myxoedema and examine the reflexes.

4 Examination of the oral cavity

Introduce yourself and gain consent for examining the patient's mouth: 'Hello, I am Dr Jones. Would it be OK if I could examine your mouth and throat?'

Clean your hands with the alcohol gel.

Ask the patient if they currently have any pain.

Ask the patient if they have dentures.

Ask the patient to open their mouth fully and say 'Ahh'. Perform a gross overview of oral cavity. Assess any restriction in the mouth opening.

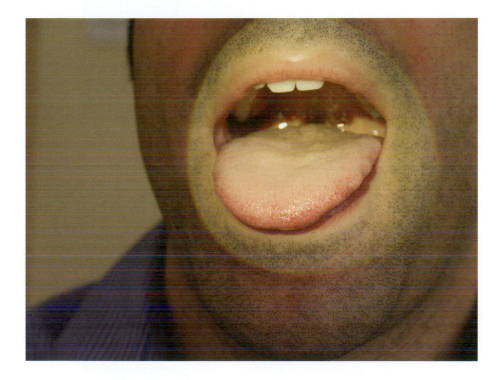

FIGURE 2.27 Examining the oral cavity, gross inspection

Using a tongue depressor, gently depress the tongue to inspect the soft palate, hard palate, uvula, tonsils and pillars.

Using two tongue blades, one in each hand, examine all teeth, gums and alveolar margins by lifting the lips away from the teeth. Start with the upper palate and then move to the lower palate.

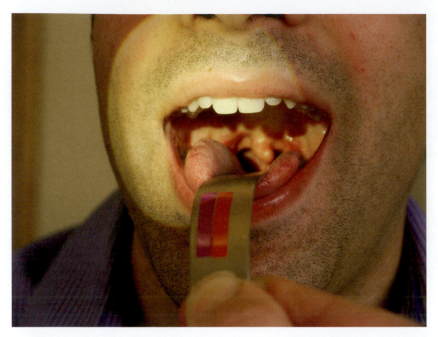

FIGURE 2.28 Use of Lack's tongue depressor to examine soft palate, hard palate, uvula, tonsils and pillars

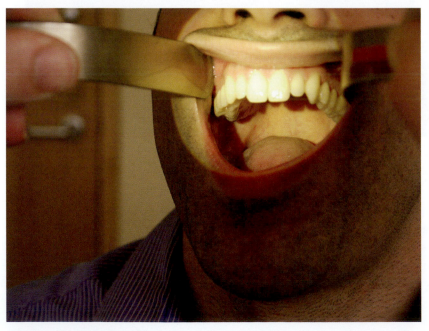

FIGURE 2.29 Use of Lack's tongue depressor to examine upper teeth, gums and alveolar margins

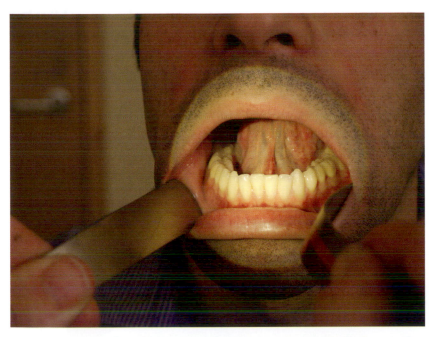

FIGURE 2.30 Use of Lack's tongue depressor to examine lower teeth, gums and alveolar margins

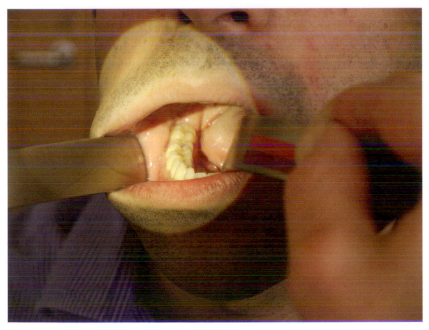

FIGURE 2.31 Use of Lack's tongue depressor to examine the buccal membranes and parotid ducts

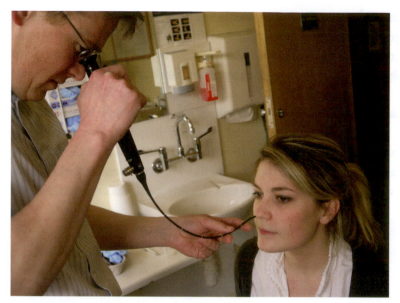

FIGURE 2.33 Flexible nasendoscopy

While visualising the larynx, ask the patient to perform three manoeuvres:
1 'say "Eee"' (to visualise adduction of vocal cords)
2 'stick your tongue out' (to visualise the valleculae)
3 'puff your cheeks out' (to visualise the pyriform fossae).

Gently withdraw the scope, reassuring the patient.

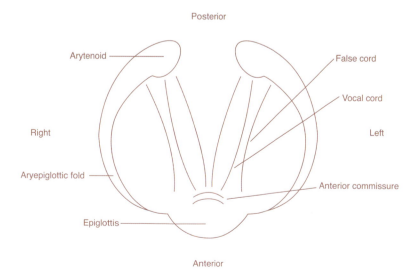

FIGURE 2.34 Diagram of the vocal tract as visualised by flexible nasendoscopy

Thank the patient and ensure they are comfortable again. Make sure you use the alcohol gel at the end.

You may be asked to draw your findings or make a drawing from a clinical photo. A schematic diagram of a normal larynx may look like Figure 2.34.

Often there is a picture with a vocal cord mass provided and you are asked to provide a labelled diagram. There are marks for labelling both the normal and the pathological areas. It is important that you can orientate (left, right, superior, inferior) correctly from the photograph. This will come with practice. In the view shown in Figure 2.34, the left cord is on the left side of the diagram. Sometimes you are shown a picture taken under direct vision, using the rigid laryngoscope. Here the cord of the left of the picture will be the right cord (as this is an inverted view of the FNE orientation that you are probably more used to).

CHAPTER 3
Communication Skills Stations

1 Consent

Stations involving taking consent for operations feature prominently in the examination. It is important to remember that you are not required to take a history. The actors will have been given some specific questions to ask the candidate. Make sure you answer these specifically, as they will certainly have marks awarded for the appropriate answer.

1.1 Grommets

TYPICAL SCENARIO

You are the ear, nose and throat (ENT) junior doctor in a busy afternoon clinic with your consultant, Mr Powell. Your consultant has seen a 5-year-old girl with her mother. He has decided that the patient needs grommets for otitis media with effusion and has asked you to explain the procedure and take consent.

Time: 7 minutes

There will be a mother present; there will not be a child in the examination. Instead, the consultation is directed at informing the mother and answering her questions.

Introduce yourself and gauge their 'starting point'.

A useful question may be: 'I understand you have just spoken to the consultant, Mr Powell, and he feels that your daughter requires an operation. The operation he has suggested is the insertion of grommets into your daughter's eardrums. Do you understand what this entails?'

This will allow you to gauge the level of information that the patient requires to make an informed choice on whether to proceed with the operation.

Start by explaining the anatomy. A diagram can be helpful at this stage. There are often 'props' available such as a model of an ear. Marks are awarded for their use, so make sure you use them if they are provided.

Explain that the ear is divided into three sections:

1   the outer ear (the part you can see)
2   the middle ear (where the bones that conduct sound are) and a tube (the Eustachian tube) that connects to the nose
3   the inner ear (where sound is made into nerve signals for the brain).

Explain the reasons for performing the operation. In this case, explain the middle ear has filled with thick fluid, or 'glue', that is not allowing the eardrum we use for hearing to move properly. Explain that we will make a hole in the eardrum to allow this fluid to drain out. We then put in a little ventilation tube (it can be helpful to draw one if one is not provided) that prevents further fluid accumulating by ventilating the middle ear. This should help the eardrum move more easily with sound and should also help the child to hear more easily.

The grommets will stay in the ear for on average 6–9 months. They tend to fall out naturally and do not need to be removed.

On the basis of the appearance of the eardrum, the child's reduced hearing (at home and on the audiogram test) and the pressure tests, it is recommended that we proceed with placing the grommets.

Explain the alternatives to surgery. In this case, explain that it is true that most children will grow out of this problem but that, unfortunately, this is a very important point in their development. Children may suffer from speech and language delay and/or behavioural problems if we do not treat them.

Explain the procedure. In this case, explain that it is a quick operation (approximately 10 minutes) that requires a short general anaesthetic (explain they will be seen by the anaesthetist later, and the anaesthetist will be able to answer any of their questions regarding this).

Explain what will happen after the operation. In this case, explain that it is advisable to keep the ears dry when washing for the first few days after the operation.

The mother may specifically ask about swimming. Advise her that this is usually permissible but that some patients may prefer to use a headband or earplugs. Diving is never advised. Explain they will be seen in clinic in about 3 months to check progress.

Explain the risks of surgery. In this case, explain that it is a safe operation but that the patient should be aware of the risks, as with any surgery.

* Infection: this is rare but is usually easily manageable with antibiotic ear drops.
* A persistent perforation ('hole in the eardrum'): sometimes this needs another operation if the hearing is affected.
* There may be a small amount of pain or bleeding, but this usually settles very quickly.

If a consent form is provided then it should be filled in with the parent. Offer to give a copy of the consent form to the patient. It is not usual that a consent form will be provided in the examination.

Ask if they have any questions. Make sure the parent has follow-up information, e.g. the clinic or ward phone number in case of concerns.

1.2 Functional endoscopic sinus surgery

TYPICAL SCENARIO

A 55-year-old man has been troubled by recurrent sinusitis for the last 10 years. Your consultant has seen the patient and has decided to perform functional endoscopic sinus surgery (FESS). The consultant has asked you to explain the procedure and to take informed consent.

Time: 7 minutes

Start by gauging the patient's starting point with a general opening statement such as: 'Perhaps you could bring me up to speed about what you've already been told about the operation.' From this you can gauge how much background information you will need to give to the patient.

Explain the anatomy of the sinuses: 'The sinuses are air- and mucus-filled spaces in the bones of the face and head. Sinusitis is an infection of these spaces. This is what has been giving you the symptoms of pain and nasal discharge. Topical treatments and antibiotics treat most sinusitis. However, in severe cases like yours this has not been able to treat it satisfactorily and an operation is required to open up draining passageways.'

Explain the reasons for performing the surgery: '"Functional endoscopic sinus surgery" is keyhole sinus surgery undertaken using a telescopic camera or "endoscope". This means we do not need to make any cuts to the outside of the face and we can do the whole operation via the nose. Ultimately, we are trying to improve the "function" of the sinuses. We will be aiming to open up the drainage pathways. This will help the flow of mucus and will stop the sinuses becoming infected. This is normally an effective procedure, although sometimes it has to be done more than once.'

Explain the alternatives to surgery: 'It would be possible to continue to have courses of antibiotics or nasal drops, but these will not combat severe chronic cases. There is also a risk of serious eye and brain infections spreading from infected sinuses. Alternative surgical approaches are more radical and involve external cuts to the face.'

Explain the procedure: 'You will require a general anaesthetic (explain the anaesthetist will answer any questions about the anaesthetic). The operation is done inside the nose without any cuts to the face. The operation usually lasts 45 minutes. After the operation you may have some nasal packing for the first 24 hours. It is common to have a blocked nose and some bloody nasal discharge for a few days after the operation.'

Explain what will happen after the operation: 'You will be able to go home the next day. We like to keep people overnight because there is a small risk of bleeding from the nose. You won't be able to go home until the nose packs have been removed. It is important not to blow your nose for the first 48 hours after the operation. Some surgeons also advise nasal douching, which means irrigating the nose with salty water. You will often need to continue using the nasal steroid sprays. You will be given instructions about this before you leave the ward.'

Explain it is routine to have 1 week off work and 2 weeks off strenuous exercise.

Explain the risks of surgery. In this case, explain that although this operation is performed regularly without any problems there are some serious risks of which they should be aware.

♦ Bleeding: it is very common to have some small quantity of bleeding from the nose and to have blood-tinged mucus for a few days after the operation.

♦ Bleeding into the eye: this is rare but can cause black eyes that will recover on their own. A more serious bleed into the eye can result if there is damage to a main artery. Although this is very rare, there is a chance that you could lose the sight in the eye. If this does happen, you may need another operation to repair the eye. In a recent survey in the UK, eye complications happened in 1 in 500 operations.

♦ Cerebrospinal fluid (CSF) leak: the sinuses lie right under the base of the brain, which is contained in special fluid called CSF. A small leak can occur via the nose if there is some bony damage. This often requires no treatment and will recover on its own. Occasionally, you may need another operation to seal over the leak. Sometimes an infection can get into the fluid that will require the use of antibiotics. CSF leaks occur in about 1 in 1000 operations.

If available, fill in the consent form with the patient. Offer to give a copy of the consent form to the patient.

Ask if they have any questions. Make sure the patient has follow-up information, e.g. the clinic or ward phone number in case of concerns.

1.3 Septoplasty

> **TYPICAL SCENARIO**
>
> You are asked to see a patient on the ward who has been admitted electively for a septoplasty. Explain the procedure to the patient and take informed consent.
>
> *Time: 7 minutes*

First off, ascertain the patient's understanding of the operation with a general open question such as: 'Can you tell me how much you have been told about the operation?'

Explain the reason for performing the operation: 'The septum is a piece of gristle inside the nose separating the left and right nostril. In most people the septum is not straight; however, in some people this can cause a blocked nostril. This operation is done to try to straighten the septum and to improve the airflow through the nose.'

Explain the alternatives to surgery: 'The operation is only undertaken when symptoms are very troubling. No harm will result from not undertaking the procedure.'

Explain the procedure: 'The operation is done through the nose and there are no cuts to the outside of the face. You shouldn't get any bruising to the face. The operation is done under general anaesthesia and you will be seen by an anaesthetist who can answer any questions about the anaesthetic. The operation takes about 45 minutes.'

Explain what will happen after the operation: 'Sometimes you will have some nasal packing, which needs to be kept in overnight. You can normally go home the next day. You will need 1 week off work and 2 weeks off strenuous exercise.'

Explain the risks of the operation: 'Septal surgery is safe surgery; however, there are some complications that of which you need to be aware.'

◀ Bleeding: we normally place 'packs' into the nose, a nasal tampon, overnight to absorb any bleeding. These will be removed before you leave the ward. It is very common to get some bloody discharge from the nose for the first couple of weeks. Larger bleeds can happen, most commonly within the first 2 weeks. On very rare occasions you might need to return to the operating theatre to stop a large bleed. There is also a chance of a blood clot or 'haematoma' forming around the wound. If this happens it is very likely that you would need to go back to theatre to have it treated.

◆ Pain: this is usually manageable with painkillers.

◆ Continued blocked nose: it will take at least 2 weeks for the nose to start feeling 'normal' again. However, we cannot guarantee alleviation of your symptoms.

◆ Change to appearance of the nose: as the septum provides support to the structure of the nose, there is a chance that the appearance of the nose can change. This is very unlikely if this is your first operation; however, with repeat operations the chances increase. In serious cases the nose can collapse.

◆ Septal perforation: there is a chance that a hole can form in the septum, causing a connection between the left and right nostrils. This often causes minimal problems such as bleeding and crusting and requires no further treatment. Ongoing perforations may need another operation to repair.

If available, fill in the consent form with the patient. Offer to give a copy of the consent form to the patient.

Ask if they have any questions. Make sure the patient has follow-up information, e.g. the clinic or ward phone number in case of concerns.

1.4 Panendoscopy and microlaryngoscopy

TYPICAL SCENARIO

A 65-year-old man has had a hoarse voice for the last 6 weeks. He is due to have a microlaryngoscopy positive/negative biopsy. Explain the procedure to him and take consent.

Time: 7 minutes

First off, ascertain the patient's starting point with a general open question such as: 'Can you tell me how much you have been told about the operations?'

Explain the reason for performing the procedure: 'We need to have a look at the voice box and the throat. We have probably already looked at the voice box in the clinic but now we need to have a better look under a general anaesthetic.

Sometimes we need to take a section of tissue so it can be examined under the microscope.'

Explain the alternatives to surgery: 'Unfortunately, if we are to best manage this condition we need to see the voice box directly by undertaking this procedure.'

Explain the procedure: 'The consultant will use a metal tube (laryngoscope and oesophagoscope) and a microscope to visualise the voice box. We will also be able to examine your nose, mouth and the rest of your throat at this time. The procedure lasts about 15 minutes.'

Explain what will happen after the procedure: 'Most patients have a sore throat after the procedure. This is usually manageable with painkillers. Some surgeons ask that you rest your voice for 24–48 hours if a biopsy has been performed. Some patients have a sore neck from the position during the operation. This usually settles without any treatment, but you should inform us if you have any long-standing neck problems. You can usually go home the same day. You will be able to eat and drink as you are able after the operation, unless the surgeon instructs differently.

Explain the risks of the procedure:

◆ Injury to lining of the throat: the risks are small but you should be aware that there is a risk of scratching the lining of the throat. This can cause some blood to come up in your saliva. If we take some tissue for a biopsy, the chances of bleeding are raised. When we are looking further down the throat (oesophagoscopy), if the damage is more severe, such as a perforation or hole in the gullet, there is a chance that you would need to stay in hospital and receive feeding through a tube through the nose until the injury has healed. It is also possible that you would need an operation to repair the perforation.

◆ Damage to teeth: there is a small risk that we can chip some teeth when we put in the metal tube. Often we use a gum guard to protect the teeth. If any damage is done we will arrange to repair the teeth at a later date.

Explain that you will see them in clinic with results.

If available, fill in the consent form with the patient. Offer to give a copy of the consent form to the patient.

Ask if they have any questions. Make sure the patient has follow-up information, e.g. the clinic or ward phone number in case of concerns.

1.5 Myringoplasty

TYPICAL SCENARIO

A 24-year-old man has a long-standing dry perforation of his right eardrum. The consultant has decided to perform a myringoplasty. Explain the procedure to the patient and take consent.

Time: 7 minutes

Start by gauging the patient's starting point.

Explain the anatomy of the ear. The use of a quick diagram here can be very useful to describe the three sections of the ear:

1   the outer ear (the part you can see)
2   the middle ear (where the bones that conduct sound are) and a tube (the Eustachian tube) that connects to the nose
3   the inner ear (where sound is made into nerve signals for the brain).

The eardrum connects the outer ear to the middle ear.

Explain the reasons for the operation: 'Most perforations are self-healing, but ones that do not heal often need an operation. The aim is to reduce the number of infections you are getting by sealing the middle ear from the outer ear. Some people notice an improvement in their hearing but we cannot guarantee this.'

Explain the alternatives to surgery: 'Without an operation the ear may continue to get infected. With this operation we hope to cut down the risks of infections and to decrease the risk of more serious infections such as meningitis.'

Explain the procedure: 'A cut is made behind the ear or above the ear hole in the crease of skin. A piece of tissue is taken from this cut. This tissue is used to repair the hole as a graft. The cut is then stitched closed and a head bandage is applied.'

Explain the risks of the operation: 'The operation has a high success rate, although it is lower if the hole is large or if you are having a lot of infections.'

◈ Failure of the operation to repair the hole in 10%–15% of cases. This may mean a further operation is required.
◈ Hearing loss: there is a small risk that the hearing can decrease or even be completely lost on the operated side.
◈ Taste disturbance: the nerve that supplies taste to the tongue runs under the

eardrum. Damage to this nerve can result in some abnormal taste on one side of the tongue. People often describe it as a metallic taste. This is usually temporary, although it can be a permanent change.

- ♦ Ringing in the ear or tinnitus: this can be temporary or permanent.
- ♦ There is a small risk that the wound can become infected; if so, this may need treatment with antibiotics.
- ♦ Dizziness: this is common for a few hours following surgery. On rare occasions, dizziness is prolonged.
- ♦ Facial paralysis: the nerve that supplies the muscles that move the face runs very close to the eardrum. Any damage to this nerve can cause a paralysis of the face; however, this is exceedingly rare in this operation. Recovery can be complete or partial.

If available, fill in the consent form with the patient. Offer to give a copy of the consent form to the patient.

Ask if they have any questions. Make sure the patient has follow-up information, e.g. the clinic or ward phone number in case of concerns.

1.6 Parotid surgery

> **TYPICAL SCENARIO**
>
> A 76-year-old man has had a unilateral swelling over his parotid gland for the last year. It has steadily increased in size. Fine needle aspiration and ultrasound has been performed that is suggestive of pleomorphic adenoma. He has been listed for a right-sided superficial parotidectomy. Explain the procedure and take consent.
>
> *Time: 7 minutes*

Start by gauging the patient's starting point.

Explain the anatomy and function of the parotid glands: 'The parotid glands are paired salivary glands on the side of the face, running from behind the ears to lie over the jaw.' (A diagram may be helpful at this stage.)

Explain the reasons for the operation: 'Parotid lumps are usually benign and not cancerous. In your case, the first tests have suggested that it is not a cancer but these lumps will carry on growing. They can begin to look very large and unattractive and there is a small chance that they can become cancerous, so we like to operate on them as soon as possible. The only way of being certain of the diagnosis is to remove the lump and send it to the laboratory.'

Explain the alternatives to surgery: 'Because of the risks previously mentioned, we like to remove this type of parotid lump; therefore, there is no alternative treatment available other than to do nothing.'

Explain the procedure: 'The operation is performed under general anaesthesia. You will see an anaesthetist who can answer any questions about the anaesthetic. The operation is done through a cut in front of the ear and down into the neck. In most people the scar heals very well.'

Explain what will happen after the operation: 'Most surgeons will insert a small drain into the neck for the first 24 hours to make sure no blood can collect in the wound. You can usually go home 48 hours after the operation or once the drain is removed and the surgeon is happy with your progress. It is advised that you take 2 weeks off work.'

Explain the risks of surgery: 'Parotid surgery is generally safe, but there are some risks that you should be aware of.'

- Facial weakness: the most serious risk is damage to the nerve that moves the facial muscles. The nerve is very closely intertwined with the gland and, although great care is taken to protect the nerve, in about 20% of people there is some weakness of the face on the operated side. In most cases this is temporary, although in about 1% of cases there is a permanent weakness.
- Numbness of the face and ear: there is some numbness to the side of the face in the majority of people and this usually recovers in time. However, often the nerve that supplies sensation to the earlobe is cut and the earlobe will be permanently numb.
- Haematoma or blood clot: bleeding under the skin can happen in about 5% of people. Occasionally this blood clot can become infected. Rarely people need to go back to theatre to stop this bleed.
- Salivary collection: in about 5% of people there can be leaking of saliva under the skin from the remaining parotid gland. This can collect in the first few weeks after surgery and needs to be drained with a needle. Usually no other treatment is required.
- Frey's syndrome: some patients find that after this surgery their cheek can become hot and sweaty while eating. This is because a nerve has grown back slightly in the wrong place. Often this will settle down with time and requires no further treatment. If symptoms are more troublesome then antiperspirant or Botox can be used.

If available, fill in the consent form with the patient. Offer to give a copy of the consent form to the patient.

Ask if they have any questions. Make sure the patient has follow-up information, e.g. the clinic or ward phone number in case of concerns.

1.7 Submandibular surgery

TYPICAL SCENARIO

A 46-year-old female is having recurrent infections of a submandibular gland secondary to a salivary gland calculus and has been placed on the list for a removal of the gland. Explain the procedure to her and take consent.

Time: 7 minutes

Start by gauging the patient's starting point

Explain the anatomy: 'The submandibular glands are two salivary glands underneath the jaw. They produce saliva when we eat. Because the saliva can be quite thick there is a chance that stones can form. These can cause infections. The aim of this operation is to remove one of the glands to stop these infections. Your ability to eat should not be affected, as there are a number of other salivary glands that can still produce saliva.'

Explain the reasons for the operation: 'In your case the duct is not draining efficiently, as it is blocked with a stone. This is causing the infections and pain.'

Explain the alternatives to surgery: 'Infections can be treated with antibiotics but an operation is needed to remove the stone.'

Explain the procedure: 'The operation is undertaken with a general anaesthetic. A cut is made under the jaw and the gland is removed.'

Explain what will happen after the operation: 'A drain will be placed into the wound for the first 24 hours after the operation. You can usually go home the next day. You will need 1 week off work.'

Explain the risks of the operation:

◈ Haematoma or blood clot can form under the skin in about 5% of people. This may require a return to the operating theatre to stop the bleed.

◈ Infection: uncommonly the wound can become infected. This is because there was infection in the gland. Sometimes pus will need to be drained from the wound and antibiotics started.

◆ Facial weakness: the nerve that makes the lower lip move runs very close to the gland. This is called the marginal mandibular branch of the facial nerve. If this is damaged it can cause a drooping of the lower lip. This can be temporary or permanent.

◆ There is a chance that the area of skin around the wound will be numb. This usually improves with time but there can be permanent changes.

◆ Numbness of tongue and changes in taste: the nerve that supplies sensation and taste to the operated side of the tongue runs very close to the nerve. Damage will cause changes that can be temporary or permanent.

◆ Injury to the nerve that 'moves' the tongue. The nerve that moves the tongue runs close to the gland. Damage to this nerve is very uncommon.

If available, fill in the consent form with the patient. Offer to give a copy of the consent form to the patient.

Ask if they have any questions. Make sure the patient has follow-up information, e.g. the clinic or ward phone number in case of concerns.

TABLE 3.1 Example mark scheme

	Yes	No	Outstanding
Shows environment considerations (e.g. suitable seating arrangement)			
Makes introduction			
Establishes rapport			
Uses appropriate non-verbal communication			
Establishes patient's understanding			
Establishes patient's level of information requirement			
Shows professionalism			
Uses appropriate terminology			
Outlines procedure			
Explains indications			
Explains important complications			
Gives information in manageable amounts			
Checks understanding			
Summarises			
Closes appropriately			
Offers follow-up, extra sources of information			

2 Explanation

These stations ask you to explain an ENT diagnosis to a patient or relative. Typical examples include a new diagnosis of benign paroxysmal positional vertigo (BPPV) and the subsequent treatment options.

It can be very helpful to use diagrams to illustrate your explanations. Usually you will be provided with relevant diagrams in the examination, although this is not always the case.

TYPICAL SCENARIO

A 48-year-old man has a new diagnosis of BPPV. Please explain the diagnosis and answer his questions.

Time: 7 minutes

Introduce yourself and confirm you are talking to the correct patient.

Start with an open question such as: 'Now, I understand you have a new diagnosis of BPPV. I was wondering if you could bring me up to speed on what you've been told about it.' This will give you the opportunity to explore the patient's current knowledge and obviously the subsequent explanation will be tailored to this.

It is useful to get a summary history from the patient as to the symptoms they are having and the time course of onset (e.g. post-traumatic BPPV occurs after head injury as opposed to the more insidious onset of idiopathic BPPV). However, the history is not the focus of this station and so you should not waste much time on history taking, as there will not be many marks on offer.

There will be marks available for exploring the **I**deas, **C**oncerns and **E**xpectations of the patient. It may be useful to ask if they have known anyone else with this condition. There may be underlying worries, e.g. a relative with vertigo who subsequently was diagnosed with a central nervous system tumour.

Move on to the explanation of the pathology. This will be aided by the use of the diagrams of the ear and semicircular canals.

Explain the ear consists of outer, middle and inner divisions and this problem involves the inner ear.

Explain that the inner ear senses balance by the position of calcium crystals. In their case, some of the crystals have moved from where they should be (utricle) to one of the canals. Hence, when they move their head the fluid shifts and causes the vertigo.

Explain the treatment is to move the head in a certain manner to realign the crystals (the Epley procedure). Explain this is an extremely effective procedure in most patients.

If they are still having problems, the procedure can be repeated. There are also vestibular rehabilitation exercises. You can offer to give them a leaflet detailing these.

Explain surgery is rarely required but is the last resort. This can involve blocking one of the semicircular canals (posterior) or cutting the balance nerves or destroying the vestibular system. However, ablative surgery runs the risk of serious complications and is by its very nature irreversible.

Ask if they have any further questions. Ensure that there are follow-up procedures in place.

TABLE 3.2 **Example mark scheme**

	Yes	No	Outstanding
Shows environmental considerations (e.g. suitable seating arrangement)			
Makes introduction			
Establishes rapport			
Uses appropriate non-verbal communication			
Establishes patient's understanding			
Establishes patient's level of information requirement			
Shows professionalism			
Asks suitable opening question			
Listens to patient's history			
Facilitates appropriately			
Summarises information and asks for clarification			
Establishes hidden agenda			
Succinct/relevant			

3 Breaking bad news

These can be potentially very difficult stations, with a number of unpredictable variables. It is important to remain calm and composed throughout the scenario, as it is easy to become flustered by outward shows of emotion from the actor, even in the artificial setting of an examination.

TYPICAL SCENARIO

Mr Jones is a 48-year-old man who has been given a diagnosis of supraglottic laryngeal cancer at his last consultant appointment. He has returned to clinic today with some questions.

Time: 7 minutes

Introduce yourself and make sure you are addressing the correct patient.

Place yourself in a non-threatening position, e.g. no barriers such as desks between you and the patient.

Ask if the patient has brought anyone with them. You can offer to bring in a nurse if they would find that helpful.

Start with an open question to gauge the starting position of the patient: 'Mr Jones, perhaps you could just bring me up to speed as to what you have been told so far.' This will guide the whole scenario. It is important to establish the patient's agenda: 'Perhaps you could give me a list of questions that you would like me to answer and I will do my best to advise you.'

Often, as in real clinic scenarios, patients cannot remember very much after hearing bad news, so it is very likely in this situation that you will need to take the explanation from the beginning.

Explain the diagnosis – always start with a 'warning shot' to prepare the patient for the news. Something like: 'I am sorry, but the news is not what we wanted to hear.' Proceed then with a clear explanation of the condition, explaining any difficult terms. A diagram is very useful here. The patient may react in a number of ways (anger, crying, bargaining). Try to remain supportive but composed. If physical contact such as a hand on the shoulder seems appropriate to you, then this can be a useful strategy to improve rapport. Always give the patient plenty of time to react (you do not need to say anything but, rather, use your body language to facilitate their reaction; this is a useful tactic for uncovering their primary concerns).

There will often be extra marks for revealing underlying concerns, e.g. 'Who will take care of my children?' These can be teased out with questions like: 'I know this is a real shock but is there anything else that you're worried about?'

Try to remain positive but do not be falsely reassuring. For example, in this instance explain there a number of treatment options open (radiotherapy, surgery, etc.).

If the patient wants to address causative factors ('Am I to blame, doctor? Was it the smoking?'), you must allow them to do this without interjecting value-laden statements. For example, here it is correct to say: 'Smoking is a known risk factor for this disease, but we can never be certain that this is the only cause.' It can be helpful at this stage to stress the treatment options.

Summarise the information you have given the patient and check that the patient understands.

Offer the patient extra sources of information (e.g. clinic phone number, details on support groups, information leaflets).

Offer to speak to the patient's relatives if they consent.

Make sure there is a follow-up plan in place.

Ask if they have any further questions.

TABLE 3.3 Example mark scheme

	Yes	No	Outstanding
Shows environmental considerations (e.g. suitable seating arrangement)			
Makes introduction			
Establishes rapport			
Uses appropriate non-verbal communication			
Establishes patient's understanding			
Establishes patient's level of information requirement			
Shows professionalism			
Ascertains if patient is accompanied			
Invites relatives/chaperone into consultation			
Gauges patient's understanding			
Gives warning shot			
Uses appropriate terminology			
Uses empathy			

(continued)

	Yes	No	Outstanding
Succinctly gives bad news			
Allows time for patient to react			
Checks understanding			
Provides a plan			
Offers to speak to family			
Offers follow-up, extra information sources			
Summarises			
Closes appropriately			

4 Discharge letter

In the examination you will often be asked to write a discharge letter to the patient's general practitioner. The majority of the marks are for including straightforward details such as the patient's name, date and type of operation. It is therefore very important not to miss these easy marks. If you have written a few discharges in your career, this should not prove too difficult a task.

In the examination you will only be provided with simple details such as the patient's name and the procedure type. Otherwise the answer paper will be blank (i.e. no *pro forma*!)

Here is an example of a discharge for a patient who has undergone a nasal polypectomy.

Example: nasal polypectomy

Paul Smith (DOB 6/1/77, Hospital No. 4234X) was admitted for endoscopic nasal polypectomy under Mr Williams for nasal polypectomy on to Ward 10 as a day case on 5 May 2011. He was discharged as planned, without complica-tion. His pre-op CT report stated: 'Patient has had ongoing nasal obstruction for 2 years. There is bilateral nasal polyposis. All other sinuses ventilated with minimal mucosal thickening.' Mr Williams will see Paul Smith in 4–6 weeks in clinic.

Answer

Patient:	Paul Smith
DOB:	6/1/77
Hospital No.:	4234X
Consultant:	Mr Williams
Ward:	10
Date of admission:	5/5/11
Date of discharge:	5/5/11
Presenting complaints:	Ongoing nasal obstruction for 2 years
Diagnosis:	Nasal polyposis
Investigations:	CT sinuses – bilateral nasal polyposis
	All other sinuses ventilated with minimal mucosal thickening
Operation:	Endoscopic nasal polypectomy
Surgeon:	Mr Williams

Complication:	No intra-operative or post-operative complications
Medications:	Given 4 weeks' saline nasal douche
	To continue with Flixonase Nasule drops 200 mcg bd
	With instructions on administration
	No other changes to medication
Advice:	All nasal packing removed before discharge
	Crusting and dry blood may cause nasal obstruction for 1–2 weeks
	Larger bleed will require readmission to hospital
	Advise 1 week off work
Follow-up:	See in clinic with histology in 4–6 weeks
Signed:	S. Jones (*sign and print name*), CT1 to Mr Williams (consultant ENT surgeon). GMC 615 4872. Contact number: 345

5 Operation note

A common question in the examination is to be asked to write an operation note for a procedure. Potentially this is a difficult station, as by its very nature it is a completely artificial situation! Rest assured the 'procedure' is usually of the nature of a tonsillectomy rather than a neck dissection.

You will only be provided with a blank sheet of paper and basic patient information:

- patient demographics including date of birth, hospital number
- date and time
- operating room
- surgeon
- anaesthetist
- type of anaesthesia
- indication for procedure
- antibiotics
- findings
- procedure/closure
- post-operative instructions
- follow-up.

Example 1: adenotonsillectomy

You have just performed an adenotonsillectomy on this patient for obstructive sleep apnoea in Theatre 2. Write the operation note.

Patient: Kieron Jones

DOB: 6/11/88

Hospital No. 1234X

Admitted as an inpatient for overnight stay under Mr Smith on 5/5/11. No intra-operative or post-operative complications were recorded. The anaesthetist was Dr Jones.

Answer

Patient:	Kieron Jones
DOB:	6/11/88
Hospital No.:	1234X

Date:	5/5/11, 2 p.m.
Theatre:	2
Anaesthetist:	Dr Jones
Surgeon:	I. Khan
Operation:	Adenotonsillectomy
Indication:	Obstructive sleep apnoea
Antibiotics:	None given
Findings:	Moderate adenoids, large grade 4 tonsils
Procedure:	Mouth gag
	Adenoids curetted
	Haemostasis with PNS pack
	Cold steel dissection of tonsils with ties to lower poles
	Diathermy at 15 W for haemostasis
	Teeth, temporomandibular joint, lips OK at end of procedure
Plan:	Airway and saturation monitoring overnight
	Watch for excessive swallowing and bleeding
	Eat and drink as able
	Regular analgesia
	Home tomorrow if no signs of bleeding
	No routine follow-up
Signed:	I. Khan (*sign and print name*), CT2 to Mr Smith (consultant ENT surgeon). GMC 6154387. Contact number: 234

Example 2: myringotomy and insertion of grommets

You have just performed bilateral myringotomies and insertion of grommets on this patient in Theatre 2 for glue ear. Write the operation note.

Patient: Damon Jones

DOB: 6/12/07

Hospital No. 1234X

Admitted as day case under Mr Smith on 6/5/11. No intra-operative or post-operative complications were recorded. The anaesthetist was Dr Jones.

Answer

Patient:	Damon Jones
DOB:	6/12/07
Hospital No.:	1234X
Date:	6/5/11, 9 a.m.
Theatre:	2
Anaesthetist:	Dr Jones
Surgeon:	T. Wilson
Operation:	Bilateral myringotomies and grommet insertion
Indication:	Bilateral glue ear
Findings:	Right – flat, dull tympanic membranes with small quantity middle ear fluid
	Left – dull tympanic membrane with large middle ear effusion
Procedure:	Ear canal suctioned of wax atraumatically
	Anterior inferior myringotomies performed
	Effusions aspirated and Shah grommets inserted
	Attics clear on right and left sides
Plan:	Routine post-operative observations
	Eat and drink as able
	Home today
	Follow-up in 2 months with audiology
	Information sheet given to patient
Signed:	T. Wilson (*sign and print name*), CT2 to Mr Smith (consultant ENT surgeon). GMC 6154387. Contact number: 234

Example 3: microlaryngoscopy and biopsy

You have just performed a microlaryngoscopy and biopsy on this patient in Theatre 2 for ongoing hoarseness. This revealed a small vocal cord polyp on R anterior ⅓ and ⅔ border. Write the operation note.

Patient: Bob Jones

DOB: 6/11/55

Hospital No. 1234X

Admitted as day case under Mr Smith on 7/5/11. No intra-operative or post-operative complications were recorded. The anaesthetist was Dr Jones.

Answer

Patient:	Bob Jones
DOB:	6/11/55
Hospital No.:	1234X
Date:	7/5/11, 11 a.m.
Theatre:	2
Anaesthetist:	Dr Jones
Surgeon:	M. Jackson
Operation:	Microlaryngoscopy and biopsy
Indication:	Hoarseness
Antibiotics:	None given
Findings:	Small vocal cord polyp on R anterior ⅓ and ⅔ border
Procedure:	Mouthguard inserted to protect teeth
	Laryngoscopy performed
	Laryngoscope in suspension
	Microscope used to inspect cords
	Microdissection of vocal cord polyp
	1:1000 adrenaline patty used for haemostasis
	Teeth, temporomandibular joint, lips clear at end of procedure
	Specimen sent to histology
Plan:	Airway and saturation monitoring
	Eat and drink as able
	24 hours' voice rest
	Home tomorrow if well
	Follow-up in 2 weeks with histology

Signed:	M. Jackson (*sign and print name*), CT2 to Mr Smith (consultant ENT surgeon). GMC 6154387. Contact number: 234

CHAPTER 4

Data and Picture Interpretation Stations

The data and picture interpretation stations make up the majority of the stations in the examination. As we stressed in the Introduction, there are some important points to remember to ensure your success with this part of the examination. First, it is important to read the question very closely and to really make sure you specifically answer what has been asked. Second, the question often asks for a list of a certain number. For example, if it asks for three causes of a condition, you will score marks only for the first three causes that you list. Remember, if the question does not directly state how many items to list it can often be inferred from the number of lines in the answer space. In the cases that follow we have not provided an exhaustive list of all possible answers but we have focused on the most important, as one should in the examination itself.

Case 1

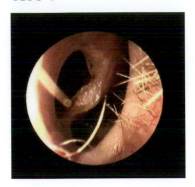

FIGURE 4.1

Q1   What is the diagnosis?

Q2   List three associated symptoms

Q3   What is the most common cause?

Q4   List four other causes

Q5   List four investigations you may perform

Q6   List three treatment options

Case 1 answers

Q1 What is the diagnosis?
Anterior nasal septal perforation

Q2 List three associated symptoms
Nasal obstruction
Crusting
Epistaxis

Q3 What is the most common cause?
Trauma (often nasal picking)

Q4 List four other causes
Previous septal surgery
Nasal cautery
Sarcoidosis
Wegener's granulomatosis

Q5 List four investigations you may perform
c-ANCA (Wegener's)
Angiotensin-converting enzyme (sarcoidosis)
Rheumatoid factor (elevated in rheumatoid arthritis, lupus, scleroderma)
Biopsy (to rule out malignancy)

Q6 List three treatment options
Nasal hygiene (saline douches, 25% glucose in glycerine)
Nasal septal prosthesis (e.g. silicone button obturator)
Surgical repair (variety of local and free flap repairs)

Case 2

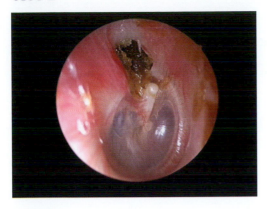

FIGURE 4.2

Q1 Describe this appearance

Q2 What type of hearing loss would be usually associated with this condition?

Q3 List four other possible symptoms

Q4 What would be the recommended treatment in a healthy 12-year-old?

Q5 List five complications you need to explain to the patient if this is left untreated

Q6 List four specific complications of surgery

Case 2 answers

Q1 Describe this appearance
Attic crust (caused by cholesteatoma)

Q2 What type of hearing loss would usually be associated with this condition?
Conductive

Q3 List four other possible symptoms
Discharge
Vertigo
Tinnitus
Facial weakness

Q4 What would be the recommended treatment in a healthy 12-year-old?
Mastoid exploration

Q5 List five complications you need to explain to the patient if this is left untreated
Deafness
Vertigo
Facial nerve palsy
Meningitis
Intracranial abscess

Q6 List four specific complications of surgery
Hearing loss
Vertigo
Facial nerve injury
Tinnitus

Case 3

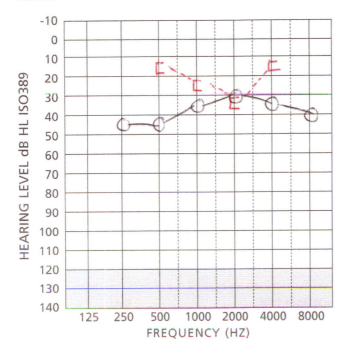

FIGURE 4.3

A 34-year-old woman presents with gradual-onset bilateral hearing loss with normal tympanic membranes.

Q1 Describe the findings on this audiogram

Q2 What is the most likely diagnosis?

Q3 List four treatment options

Q4 What other audiometric investigation would you perform?

Case 3 answers

Q1 Describe the findings on this audiogram
Right conductive hearing loss with Carhart's notch (narrowing of air-bone gap at 2000 Hz)

Q2 What is the most likely diagnosis?
Otosclerosis

Q3 List four treatment options
Observation
Fluoride
Hearing aid
Stapedectomy

Q4 What other audiometric investigation would you perform?
Tympanometry – typically shows an A_s curve (shallow peak at approximately 0 daPa)

Case 4

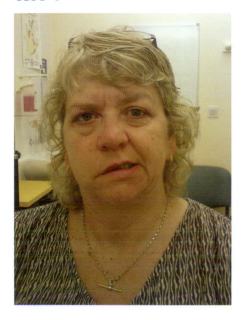

FIGURE 4.4

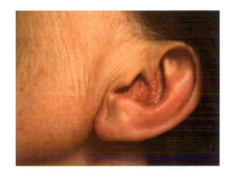

FIGURE 4.4A

A 60-year-old woman presents with facial weakness and a rash.

Q1 What is the likely diagnosis?

Q2 What is the aetiology?

Q3 List four associated symptoms

Q4 List four treatment options

Q5 List three audiometric tests for this condition

Q6 Name a serological test for this condition

Q7 How does the prognosis compare with an idiopathic cause (Bell's palsy)?

Case 4 answers

Q1 What is the likely diagnosis?
Herpes zoster oticus (Ramsay Hunt syndrome)

Q2 What is the aetiology?
Varicella zoster infection

Q3 List four associated symptoms
Otalgia
Hearing loss
Pharyngeal ulceration
Other cranial neuropathies

Q4 List four treatment options
Analgesia
Eye care, e.g eye taping and artificial tears
Corticosteroids
Aciclovir

Q5 List three audiometric tests for this condition
Pure-tone audiogram
Acoustic reflexes
Electroneurography

Q6 Name a serological test for this condition
Varicella zoster IgG

Q7 How does the prognosis compare with an idiopathic cause (Bell's palsy)?
The prognosis is poor in comparison with Bell's palsy

Case 5

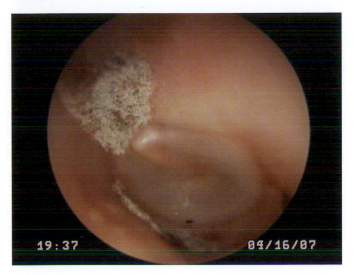

19:37   04/16/07

FIGURE 4.5

Q1 What is the diagnosis?

Q2 List two possible causative organisms

Q3 List four predisposing factors

Q4 List four components of the management

Case 5 answers

Q1 What is the diagnosis?
Fungal otitis externa/otomycosis

Q2 List two possible causative organisms
Aspergillus niger
Candida albicans
Actinomyces

Q3 List four predisposing factors
Topical antibiotics
Water exposure
Canal trauma
Diabetes

Q4 List four components of the management
Aural toilet
Topical antifungal, e.g. clotrimazole
Water precautions
Analgesia

Case 6

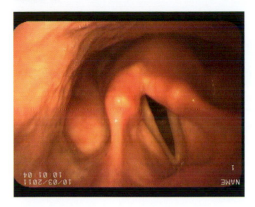

FIGURE 4.6

The flexible nasendoscopy view of the cords is of a 45-year-old man with a weak voice. You have asked him to attempt to vocalise.

Q1 Describe the abnormality

Q2 List two investigations you would request to determine the aetiology

Q3 List two treatment options to improve voice quality if this is found to be idiopathic

Case 6 answers

Q1 Describe the abnormality
Failure of medialisation of left vocal cord/left vocal cord palsy

Q2 List two investigations you would request to determine the aetiology
Chest X-ray (CXR)
Computed tomography (CT) of the skull base to mediastinum

Q3 List two treatment options to improve voice quality if this is found to be idiopathic
Speech and language therapy
Surgery to medialise affected vocal cord

Case 7

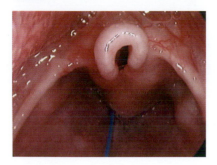

FIGURE 4.7

A 2-month-old boy presents to A&E with difficult, noisy breathing.

Q1   What is the diagnosis?

Q2   What is the classic description of the pathology shown in the picture?

Q3   List two presenting signs

Q4   List two investigations you may perform

Q5   List three treatment options

Case 7 answers

Q1 What is the diagnosis?
Laryngomalacia

Q2 What is the classic description of the pathology shown in the picture?
Omega-shaped epiglottis

Q3 List two presenting signs
Harsh inspiratory noises/stridor
Mild tachypnoea

Q4 List two investigations you may perform
Laryngotracheobronchoscopy
Polysomnography

Q5 List three treatment options
Conservative
Oxygen administration
Surgery: supraglottoplasty, rarely tracheostomy

Case 8

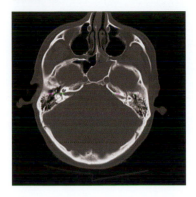

FIGURE 4.8

A 24-year-old man presents with hearing loss following a road traffic accident.

Q1   What is this study?

Q2   What is the abnormality?

Q3   Describe what the pure-tone audiogram would very likely show

Q4   Will the patient's hearing recover?

Q5   List five other symptoms the patient may experience

Case 8 answers

Q1   What is this study?
Axial CT of left temporal bone

Q2   What is the abnormality?
Transverse fracture, left temporal bone

Q3   Describe what the pure-tone audiogram would very likely show
Left-sided sensorineural deafness/dead ear

Q4   Will the patient's hearing recover?
No

Q5   List five other symptoms the patient may experience
Vertigo
Facial palsy
Cerebrospinal fluid (CSF) leak
Conductive hearing loss
Tinnitus

Case 9

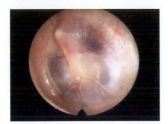

FIGURE 4.9

Q1 Describe two abnormal features

Q2 Draw and describe the associated tympanogram

Q3 Describe the expected pure-tone audiogram

Q4 List four management options

Q5 List two sequelae

Case 9 answers

Q1 Describe two abnormal features
Retracted tympanic membrane
Fluid behind tympanic membrane

Q2 Draw and describe the associated tympanogram
A flat trace. This is an example tympanogram from a 4-year-old child with Eustachian tube dysfunction.

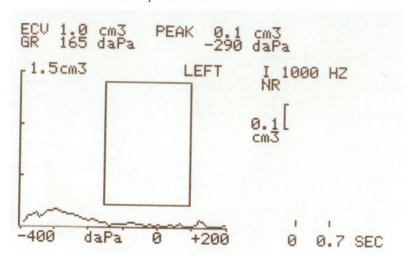

FIGURE 4.9A

Q3 Describe the expected pure-tone audiogram
Conductive hearing loss, particularly at low frequencies

Q4 List four management options
Watchful waiting
Hearing aid
Grommets
Adenoidectomy

Q5 List two sequelae
Speech and language delay
Acute otitis media (AOM)

Case 10

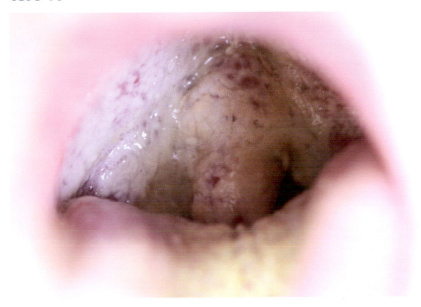

FIGURE 4.10

Q1 What is the diagnosis?

Q2 List three treatments associated with this appearance

Q3 List two diseases associated with this appearance

Q4 List two management strategies

Case 10 answers

Q1   What is the diagnosis?
Oral candidiasis

Q2   List three treatments associated with this appearance
Systemic/inhaled corticosteroids
Systemic antibiotics
Chemotherapy/radiotherapy

Q3   List two diseases associated with this appearance
Diabetes
Acquired immune deficiency syndrome

Q4   List two management strategies
Oral antifungal, e.g. nystatin
Oral hygiene

Case 11

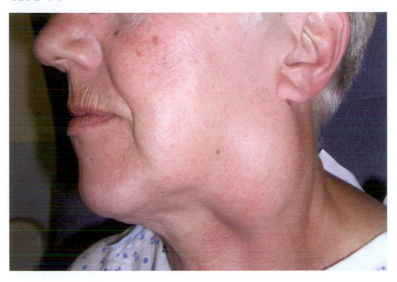

FIGURE 4.11

Q1   In which anatomical triangle of the neck is the lesion in the photograph?

Q2   What are the four most likely diagnoses?

Q3   List three tests that could help distinguish among the possible diagnoses

Q4   If the lesion turned out to be cystic, what would be your treatment options?

Q5   What is the embryological origin of a cystic lesion in this area?

Case 11 answers

Q1 In which anatomical triangle of the neck is the lesion in the photograph?
Left anterior triangle

Q2 What are the four most likely diagnoses?
Infective lymphadenopathy
Branchial cyst
Lymphoma
Metastatic cancer

Q3 List three tests that could help distinguish among the possible diagnoses
Fine needle aspiration (FNA; reactive, neoplastic cells, cholesterol-rich fluid in the case of branchial cysts)
Ultrasound scan (USS; differentiate between neoplastic and reactive lymph nodes/cysts)
Bloods including full blood count (FBC) and c-reactive protein (e.g. to detect infective process)

Q4 If the lesion turned out to be cystic, what would be your treatment options?
Treat any underlying infection, surgical removal of cyst and send for histology

Q5 What is the embryological origin of a cystic lesion in this area?
From the second branchial cleft

Case 12

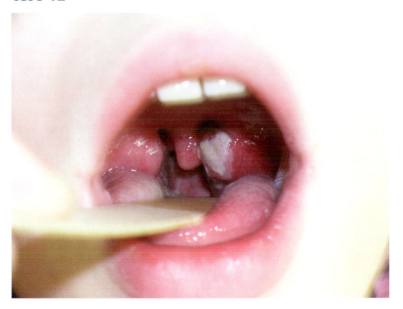

FIGURE 4.12

Q1   What is the diagnosis?

Q2   Describe three key steps in managing this patient

Q3   Name one specific test you would perform

Q4   What antibiotic would you not prescribe in this case?

Q5   List five indications for tonsillectomy

Case 12 answers

Q1   What is the diagnosis?
Tonsillitis

Q2   Describe three key steps in managing this patient
Analgesia and antipyretics
Antibiotics, e.g. intravenous benzyl penicillin
Intravenous fluid resuscitation

Q3   Name one specific test you would perform
Monospot/Paul–Bunnell test for glandular fever

Q4   What antibiotic would you not prescribe in this case?
Amoxicillin (due to type IV hypersensitivity reaction presenting as a rash)

Q5   List five indications for tonsillectomy
Recurrent severe tonsilitis for over 1 year:
- seven or more well-documented, clinically significant, adequately treated sore throats in the preceding year or
- five or more such episodes in each of the preceding 2 years or
- three or more such episodes in each of the preceding 3 years.

Treatment of obstructive sleep apnoea
Diagnosis of tonsillar malignancy in cases of unilateral enlarged tonsil
Recurrent quinsy
Treatment of snoring

Case 13

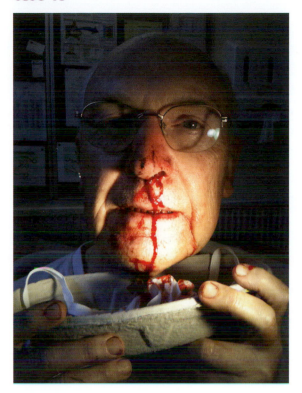

FIGURE 4.13

Q1 What is the diagnosis?

Q2 Describe three key steps in managing this patient

Q3 List three specific causes/precipitants for this complaint

Q4 Name the arteries supplying the nasal septum

Case 13 answers

Q1 What is the diagnosis?
Anterior epistaxis

Q2 Describe three key steps in managing this patient
Control bleeding using first aid, nasal cautery and nasal packing
Intravenous access for intravenous fluid therapy and bloods, including FBC
Surgical intervention for recalcitrant bleeding, e.g. sphenopalatine artery ligation

Q3 List three specific causes/precipitants for this complaint
Trauma
Anticoagulation
Hypertension

Q4 Name the arteries supplying the nasal septum
Blood supply from the internal and external carotid arteries
Sphenopalatine artery and greater palatine artery (from the maxillary artery, a branch of the external carotid)
Anterior ethmoidal artery (from the ophthalmic artery from the internal carotid)
Branches of the facial artery (from the external carotid)

Case 14

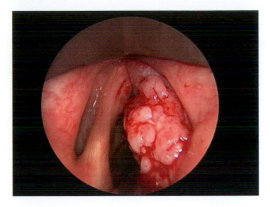

FIGURE 4.14

Q1   Describe the clinical photograph

Q2   Typically, how do patients with this type of lesion present?

Q3   List two risk factors

Q4   Name the staging system currently in use

Q5   List two investigations you would perform

Q6   List three management strategies

Case 14 answers

Q1 Describe the clinical photograph
Ulcerative growth from right vocal cord

Q2 Typically, how do patients with this type of lesion present?
Hoarse voice
Stridor in severe cases

Q3 List two risk factors
Smoking
Excess alcohol consumption

Q4 Name the staging system currently in use
Tumour node metastasis

Q5 List two investigations you would perform
CT of the head, neck and chest
Microlaryngoscopy and biopsy

Q6 List three management strategies
Surgery
Chemotherapy/radiotherapy
Palliation

Case 15

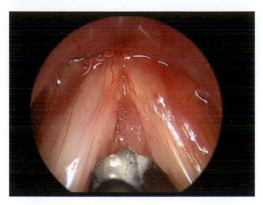

FIGURE 4.15

This 6-year-old girl has a recurrent lesion of the vocal cords.

Q1   Describe the clinical photograph

Q2   Typically, how do children with this type of lesion present?

Q3   How would you manage this patient?

Q4   What is the causative agent?

Q5   Would you consider a tracheostomy in this patient?

Case 15 answers

Q1 Describe the clinical photograph
Papilloma of the anterior commissure of the larynx

Q2 Typically, how do children with this type of lesion present?
Hoarse voice
Stridor in severe cases

Q3 How would you manage this patient?
Microlaryngoscopy
Microdebridement/laser ablation

Q4 What is the causative agent?
Human papillomavirus (types 6 and 11)

Q5 Would you consider a tracheostomy in this patient?
Tracheostomy should only be used as a last resort, as it increases the chance
of disease spreading distally

Case 16

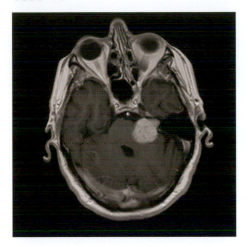

FIGURE 4.16

Q1 What type of scan is this?

Q2 What is the most obvious abnormality?

Q3 What is the most likely diagnosis?

Q4 List three typical ways these lesions present

Q5 List three treatment modalities

Q6 List three alternative diagnoses

Case 16 answers

Q1 What type of scan is this?
Magnetic resonance imaging with gadolinium enhancement

Q2 What is the most obvious abnormality?
Right cerebellopontine angle lesion

Q3 What is the most likely diagnosis?
Acoustic neuroma

Q4 List three typical ways these lesions present
Unilateral hearing loss
Unilateral tinnitus
Other cranial neuropathies, e.g. sensation changes in V nerve distribution

Q5 List three treatment modalities
Conservative (watch-and-wait approach)
Surgery
Stereotactic radiosurgery

Q6 List three alternative diagnoses
Meningioma
Cholesterol granuloma
Facial schwannoma

Case 17

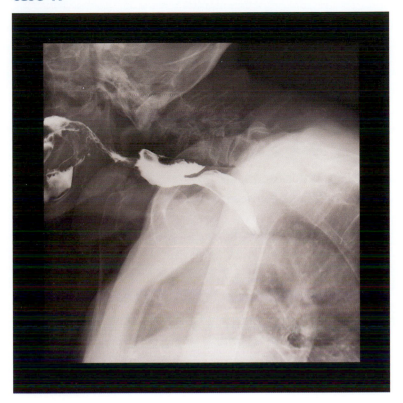

FIGURE 4.17

Q1   What is the diagnosis?

Q2   List four ways this would typically present

Q3   What is the aetiology of this condition?

Q4   List three treatment options

Case 17 answers

Q1 What is the diagnosis?
Pharyngeal pouch

Q2 List four ways this would typically present
Regurgitation
Dysphagia
Weight loss
Halitosis

Q3 What is the aetiology of this condition?
Natural weakness at Killian's dehiscence between inferior constrictor and cricopharyngeus

Q4 List three treatment options
Conservative
Endoscopic stapling
Open surgical excision

Case 18

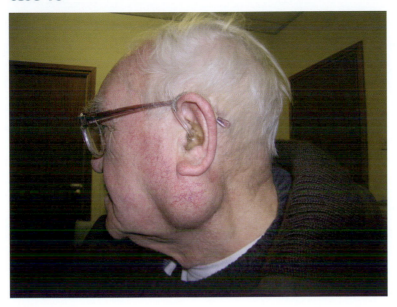

FIGURE 4.18

Q1 What is the abnormality pictured here?

Q2 Name two common tumours in this gland

Q3 List two symptoms that would concern you about malignancy

Q4 List two investigations you would perform

Q5 List three things you would warn the patient about if you were considering surgical removal of the lump

Case 18 answers

Q1   What is the abnormality pictured here?
Left parotid lump

Q2   Name two common tumours in this gland
Pleomorphic adenoma
Warthin's tumour

Q3   List two symptoms that would concern you about malignancy
Facial nerve palsy
Pain

Q4   List two investigations you would perform
FNA
Imaging, e.g. CT

Q5   List three things you would warn the patient about if you were considering surgical removal of the lump
Bleeding/haematoma formation
Facial nerve injury
Frey's syndrome (gustatory sweating)

Case 19

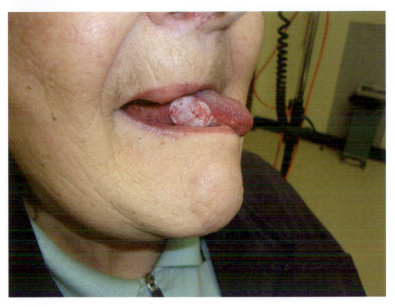

FIGURE 4.19

Q1 What is the most likely diagnosis?

Q2 List three risk factors

Q3 List two investigations you would perform

Q4 List three management strategies

Case 19 answers

Q1   What is the most likely diagnosis?
Right-sided tongue squamous cell carcinoma

Q2   List three risk factors
Smoking
Excessive alcohol consumption
Betel nut chewing

Q3   List two investigations you would perform
Staging CT of the head, neck, chest
Panendoscopy and biopsy

Q4   List three management strategies
Surgery
Chemotherapy/radiotherapy
Palliation

Case 20

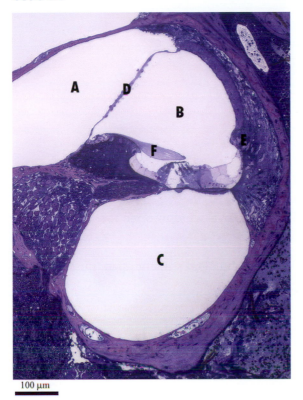

100 μm

FIGURE 4.20

Q1   Name the structures labelled A–F

Q2   What is the major cation in A?

Q3   Which compartment (A–F) does the oval window open to?

Q4   Name the point where the scala vestibuli and scala tympani meet

Q5   What is the modiolus?

Q6   Which compartment is involved in Ménière's syndrome?

Case 20 answers

Q1 Name the structures labelled A–F
A: scala vestibuli
B: scala media
C: scala tympani
D: Reissner's membrane
E: stria vascularis
F: tectorial membrane

Q2 What is the major cation in A?
Sodium

Q3 Which compartment (A–F) does the oval window open to?
A

Q4 Name the point where the scala vestibuli and scala tympani meet
Helicotrema

Q5 What is the modiolus?
The conical-shaped central axis of the cochlea

Q6 Which compartment is involved in Ménière's syndrome?
B

Case 21

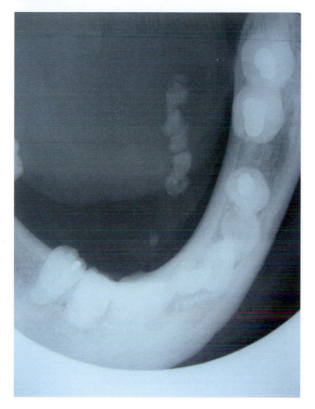

FIGURE 4.21

Q1   What is this imaging modality?

Q2   What is the obvious abnormality?

Q3   List three treatment options

Q4   List three specific complications of surgery to the gland

Case 21 answers

Q1   What is this imaging modality?
Plain X-ray of the floor of mouth

Q2   What is the obvious abnormality?
Left submandibular salivary duct stone

Q3   List three treatment options
Symptomatic, e.g. increased fluid intake and analgesia
Sialoendoscopy and basket retrieval of stone
Surgical removal of gland

Q4   List three specific complications of surgery to the gland
Weakness of lip (damage to marginal mandibular nerve)
Taste disturbance
Weakness of tongue

Case 22

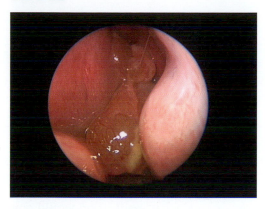

FIGURE 4.22

This is a photograph from an endoscopic intranasal operation.

Q1   What is the diagnosis?

Q2   List two presenting symptoms

Q3   List two medical treatments

Q4   If this patient also reported 'a wheezy chest', what medication would you advise them to avoid?

Q5   List three main complications of surgical removal

Case 22 answers

Q1   What is the diagnosis?
Nasal polyp

Q2   List two presenting symptoms
Nasal obstruction
Anosmia

Q3   List two medical treatments
Intranasal steroids
Systemic steroids

Q4   If this patient also reported 'a wheezy chest', what medication would you advise them to avoid?
Aspirin (this may represent Samter's triad)

Q5   List three main complications of surgical removal
Bleeding
Risk to vision
CSF leak

Case 23

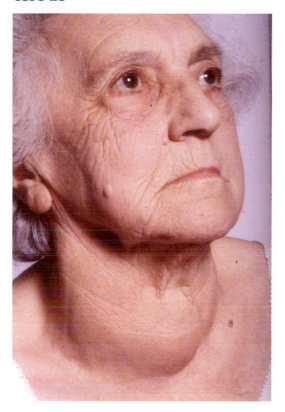

FIGURE 4.23

Thyroid-stimulating hormone, 23 (0.4–3.0)
Free T4, 1.1 (0.8–1.8)
Total T3, 159 (80–180)
Thyroglobulin, 28 (<35)
Thyroid peroxidase antibodies, 675 (<45)

Q1   What is the diagnosis?

Q2   List two tests to help confirm the diagnosis

Q3   List five typical presenting symptoms of hypothyroidism

Q4   Name the most common medical treatment

Q5   What are two indications for surgery?

Case 23 answers

Q1 What is the diagnosis?
Hashimoto's thyroiditis

Q2 List two tests to help confirm the diagnosis
USS
FNA

Q3 List five typical presenting symptoms of hypothroidism
Weight gain
Voice change
Loss of hair
Cold intolerance
Muscle weakness

Q4 Name the most common medical treatment
Thyroid hormone replacement

Q5 What are two indications for surgery?
Any risk of malignancy
Mass effect causing airway compromise

Case 24

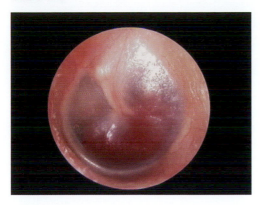

FIGURE 4.24

Q1   What is the abnormality pictured here?

Q2   List two presenting symptoms

Q3   What is the staging system used?

Q4   What is the tissue of origin of this lesion?

Q5   List three management strategies

Case 24 answers

Q1   What is the abnormality pictured here?
        Glomus tympanicum

Q2   List two presenting symptoms
        Conductive hearing loss
        Pulsatile tinnitus

Q3   What is the staging system used?
        Fisch classification

Q4   What is the tissue of origin of this lesion?
        Neuroendocrine tissue

Q5   List three management strategies
        Observation with repeat scanning
        Stereotactic radiosurgery
        Surgical resection

Case 25

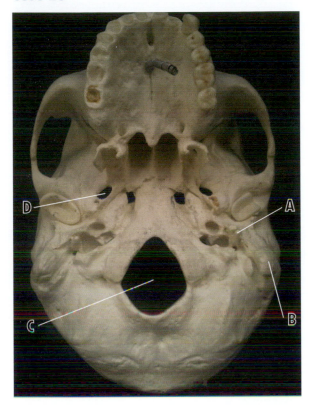

FIGURE 4.25

Q1   What is the structure labelled A? Name a ligament and a muscle that attaches here

Q2   What is the structure labelled B? List two muscles that attach here

Q3   What is the structure labelled C? List four structures that pass through this structure

Q4   What is the structure labelled D? Name a structure that passes through this structure

Case 25 answers

Q1   What is the structure labelled A? Name a ligament and a muscle that attaches here
Styloid process
Styloglossus muscle
Stylohyoid ligament

Q2   What is the structure labelled B? List two muscles that attach here
Mastoid process
Sternocleidomastoid
Posterior belly of digastric

Q3   What is the structure labelled C? List four structures that pass through this structure
Foramen magnum, spinal cord
Meninges
Vertebral arteries
Spinal root of cranial nerve XI

Q4   What is the structure labelled D? Name a structure that passes through this structure
Foramen ovale
Mandibular division of cranial nerve V

Case 26

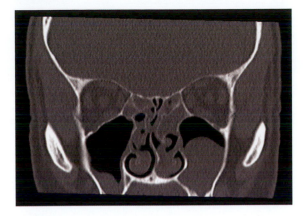

FIGURE 4.26

Q1 What is this investigation?

Q2 What are the abnormalities shown?

Q3 List three typical symptoms this patient may present with

Q4 List five risks of endoscopic surgery for this condition

Q5 If damaged, which vessel can cause a rise in intraorbital pressure?

Case 26 answers

Q1 What is this investigation?
CT paranasal sinuses

Q2 What are the abnormalities shown?
Opacification of the right maxillary and ethmoid sinuses

Q3 List three typical symptoms this patient may present with
Rhinorrhea
Nasal obstruction
Anosmia

Q4 List five risks of endoscopic surgery for this condition
Bleeding
Infection
Damage to vision
CSF leak
Meningitis

Q5 If damaged, which vessel can cause a rise in intraorbital pressure?
Anterior ethmoidal artery

Case 27

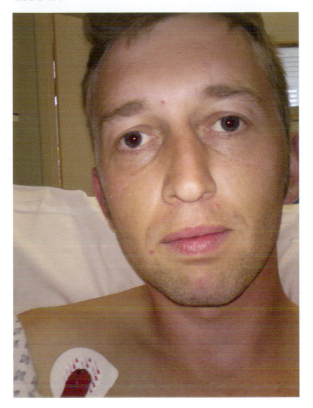

FIGURE 4.27

Q1 What the obvious pathology?

Q2 What is your advice to the referring A&E officer?

Q3 What is the management if this patient is not seen until 3 months after the injury?

Case 27 answers

Q1 What the obvious pathology?
Fractured nasal bones

Q2 What is your advice to the referring A&E officer?
If no other injuries, no septal haematoma and no ongoing epistaxis, the patient can be seen in the ENT clinic in 1 week when the swelling has subsided

Q3 What is the management if this patient is not seen until 3 months after the injury?
It is most likely that the bones will have healed and, therefore, will need a septorhinoplasty under general anaesthesia

Case 28

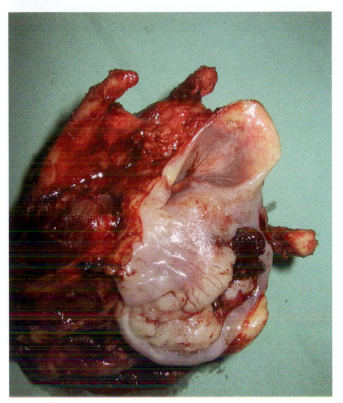

FIGURE 4.28

Q1 What is the obvious pathology?

Q2 List four ways the patient may have presented

Q3 What is the staging system currently in use?

Q4 List three treatment modalities

Case 28 answers

Q1 What the obvious pathology?
Right pyriform fossa ulcerative lesion

Q2 List four ways the patient may have presented
Weight loss
Dysphagia
Odynophagia
Referred otalgia

Q3 What is the staging system currently in use?
Tumour node metastasis

Q4 List three treatment modalities
Surgery
Chemotherapy/radiotherapy
Palliation

Case 29

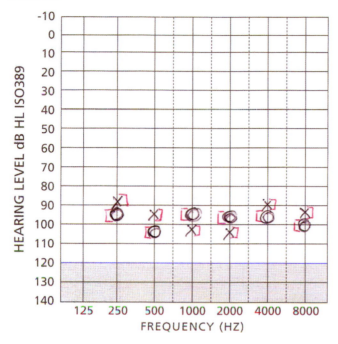

FIGURE 4.29 A

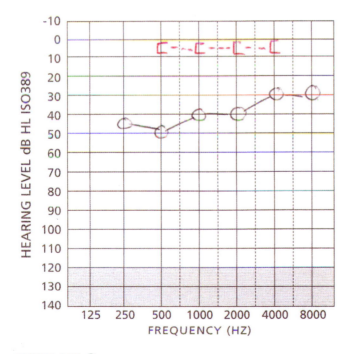

FIGURE 4.29 B

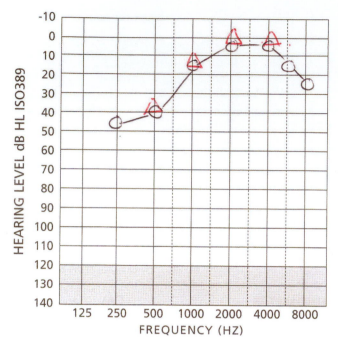

FIGURE 4.29 C

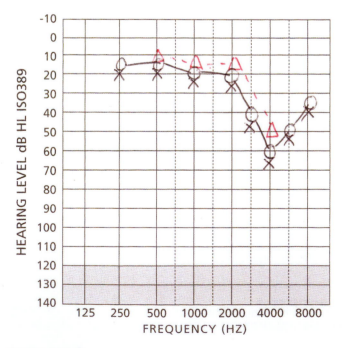

FIGURE 4.29 D

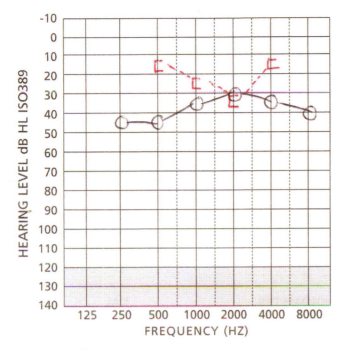

FIGURE 4.29 E

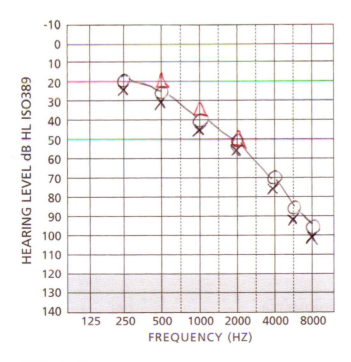

FIGURE 4.29 F

Q1 Which audiogram best fits with glue ear?

Q2 Which audiogram best fits with otosclerosis?

Q3 Which audiogram best fits with presbycusis?

Q4 Which audiogram would benefit most from cochlear implantation?

Q5 Which audiogram best fits with noise-induced hearing loss?

Q6 Which audiogram best fits with Ménière's syndrome?

Case 29 answers

Q1 Which audiogram best fits with glue ear?
B

Q2 Which audiogram best fits with otosclerosis?
E

Q3 Which audiogram best fits with presbycusis?
F

Q4 Which audiogram would benefit most from cochlear implantation?
A

Q5 Which audiogram best fits with noise-induced hearing loss?
D

Q6 Which audiogram best fits with Ménière's syndrome?
C

Case 30

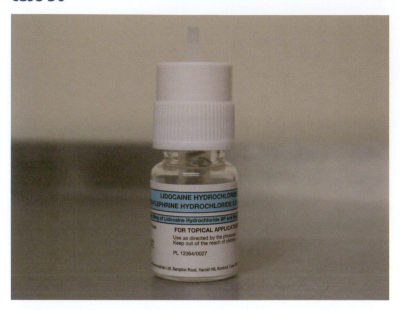

FIGURE 4.30 A

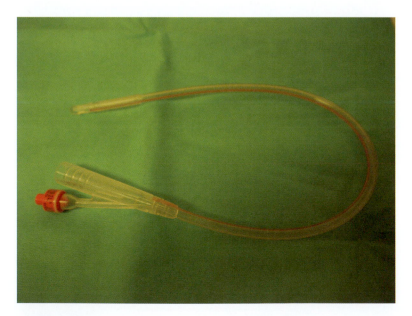

FIGURE 4.30 B

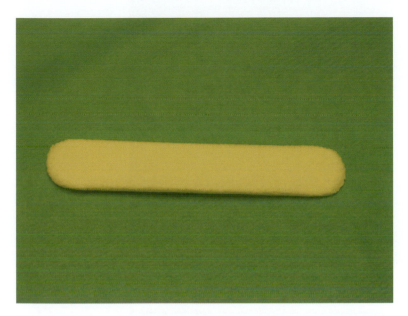

FIGURE 4.30 **C**

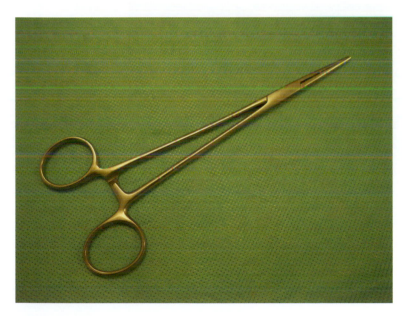

FIGURE 4.30 **D**

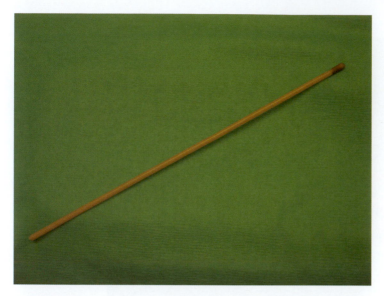

FIGURE 4.30 E

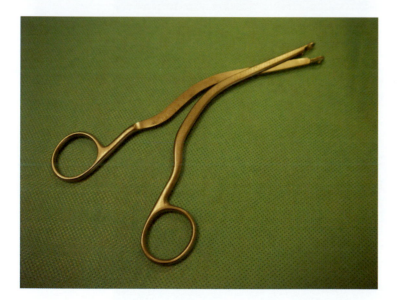

FIGURE 4.30 F

Q1 List four objects used in the management of epistaxis

Q2 Name object D

Q3 Name object F

Q4 What does the acronym BIPP stand for?

Case 30 answers

Q1 List four objects used in the management of epistaxis
A, B, C and E

Q2 Name object D
Birkett straight forceps

Q3 Name object F
Tonsil grasping forceps

Q4 What does the acronym BIPP stand for?
Bismuth, iodoform and paraffin paste

Case 31

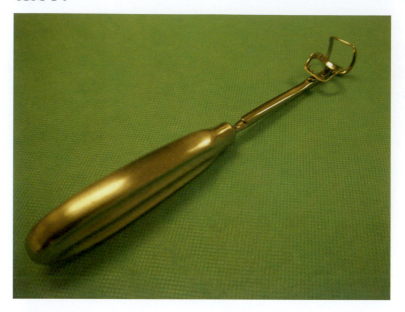

FIGURE 4.31 A

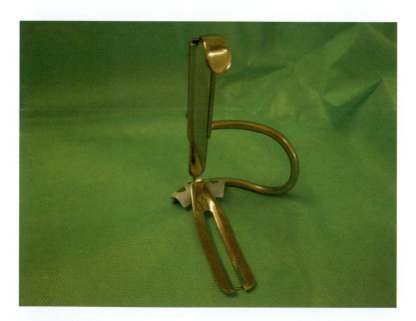

FIGURE 4.31 B

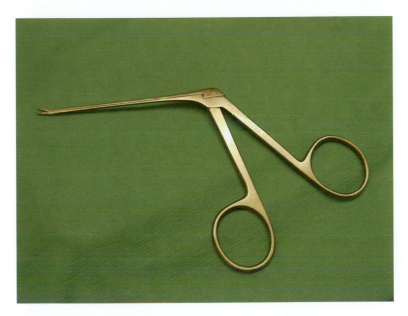

FIGURE 4.31 C

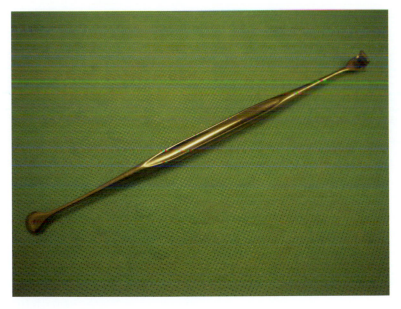

FIGURE 4.31 D

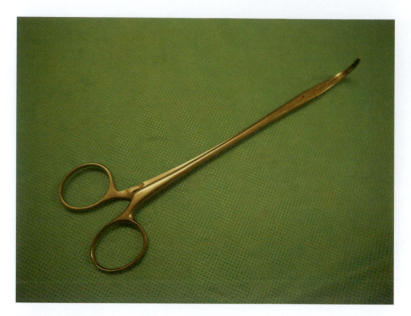

FIGURE 4.31 E

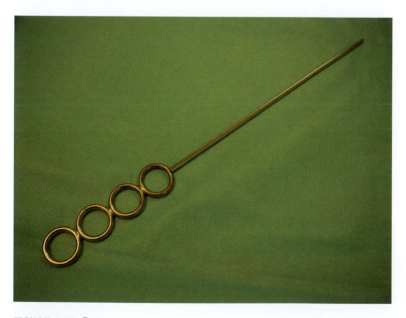

FIGURE 4.31 F

Q1   List four objects used in tonsillectomy

Q2   Name object B

Q3   Name object D

Q4   Name object F

Case 31 answers

Q1 List four objects used in tonsillectomy
B, D, E and F

Q2 Name object B
Boyle–Davis gag

Q3 Name object D
Mollison pillar retractor

Q4 Name object F
Draffin rod

Case 32

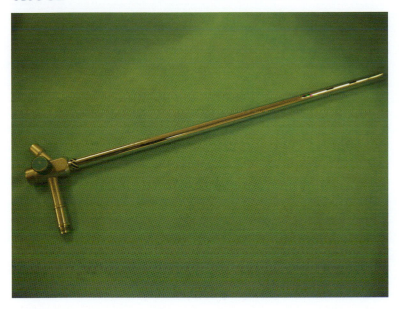

FIGURE 4.32 A

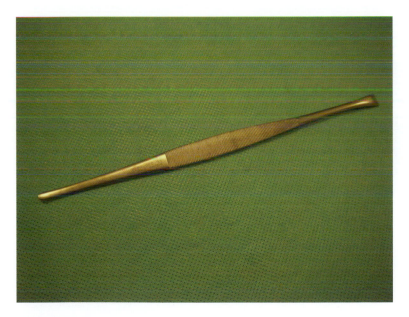

FIGURE 4.32 B

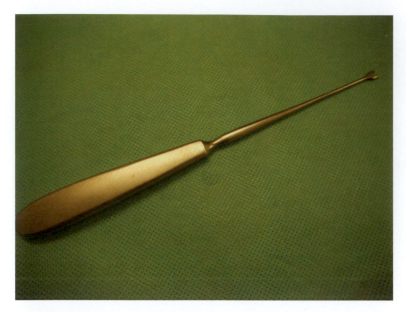

FIGURE 4.32 C

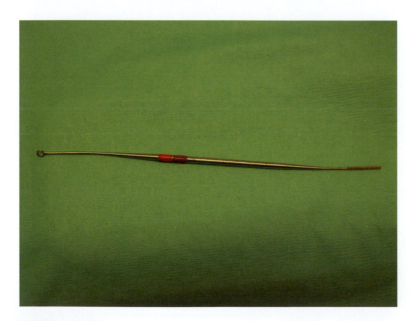

FIGURE 4.32 D

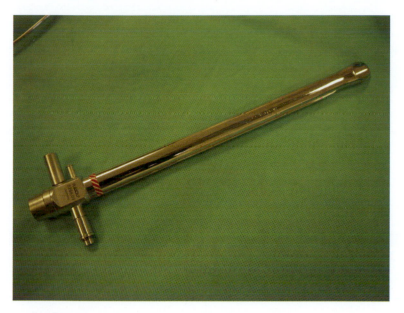

FIGURE 4.32 E

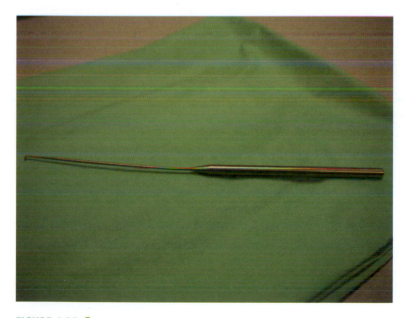

FIGURE 4.32 F

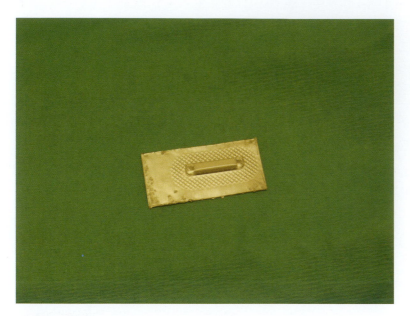

FIGURE 4.32 G

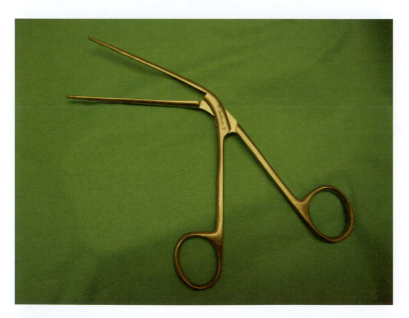

FIGURE 4.32 H

Q1 Which instrument is most appropriately used to remove an inhaled foreign body?

Q2 Which instrument is most appropriately used to remove an oesophageal foreign body?

Q3 Which instruments are most appropriately used to remove a foreign body from an ear?

Q4 Name object G

Case 32 answers

Q1 Which instrument is most appropriately used to remove an inhaled foreign body?
A

Q2 Which instrument is most appropriately used to remove an oesophageal foreign body?
B

Q3 Which instruments are most appropriately used to remove a foreign body from an ear?
D and F

Q4 Name object G
Pope wick

Case 33

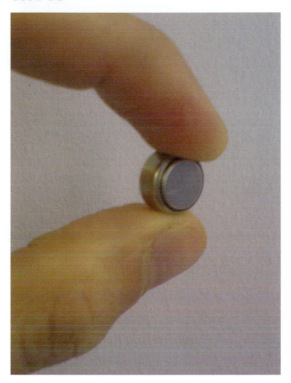

FIGURE 4.33

Q1   What is this?

Q2   What is its most common use in ENT?

Q3   List two consequences of this being inserted into the nasal cavity

Q4   List two consequences of this being inserted into the ear of a child

Q5   List three investigations you would perform for an adult with learning disabilities reported to have ingested this 2 hours ago

Q6   If presence were confirmed at the level of the cricopharyngeus, what would you do?

Q7   What is the most serious risk of this procedure?

Case 33 answers

Q1 What is this?
Watch battery

Q2 What is its most common use in ENT?
Hearing aid

Q3 List two consequences of this being inserted into the nasal cavity
Acid burn to nasal mucosa
Septal perforation

Q4 List two consequences of this being inserted into the ear of a child
Acid burn to external auditory canal
Deafness

Q5 List three investigations you would perform for an adult with learning disabilities reported to have ingested this 2 hours ago
Erect CXR
Lateral soft tissue neck X-ray
Abdominal X-ray

Q6 If presence were confirmed at the level of the cricopharyngeus, what would you do?
Urgent rigid oesophagoscopy for removal

Q7 What is the most serious risk of this procedure?
Perforated oesophagus

Case 34

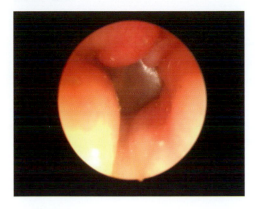

FIGURE 4.34

Q1 What is the abnormality pictured here?

Q2 List two associated symptoms

Q3 What is the most common aetiology?

Q4 List two management strategies

Q5 Name one measure the patient could take to prevent progression

Case 34 answers

Q1   What is the abnormality pictured here?
Bony exostoses of the auditory canal

Q2   List two associated symptoms
Deafness
Wax impaction

Q3   What is the most common aetiology?
Cold-water exposure

Q4   List two management strategies
No treatment if asymptomatic
Surgical bony meatoplasty

Q5   Name one measure the patient could take to prevent progression
Use earplugs when swimming

Case 35

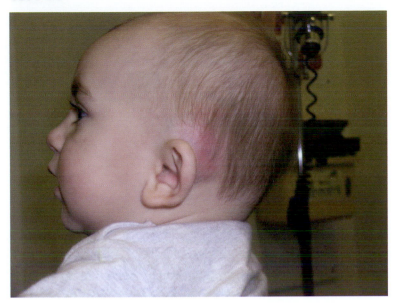

FIGURE 4.35

Q1   What is the abnormality pictured here?

Q2   List three presenting symptoms

Q3   What is the most common aetiology?

Q4   List two management options

Q5   List three complications that can occur as a result of this condition

Case 35 answers

Q1 What is the abnormality pictured here?
Left acute mastoiditis

Q2 List three presenting symptoms
Otalgia
Fever
Ear discharge

Q3 What is the most common aetiology?
AOM

Q4 List two management options
Intravenous antibiotics
Cortical mastoidectomy

Q5 List three complications that can occur as a result of this condition
Sigmoid sinus thrombosis
Intracranial abscess
Meningitis

Index

Entries in **bold** refer to figures or tables.